W9-CDC-121

NURSING EDUCATION
Practical Methods and Models

Barbara J. Brown, R.N., Ed.D., F.A.A.N.
Peggy L. Chinn, R.N., Ph.D., F.A.A.N.
Editors

A collection of articles from Nursing Administration Quarterly and Advances in Nursing Science

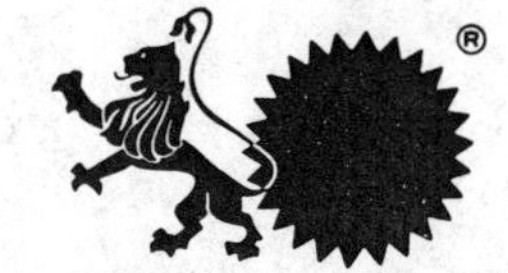

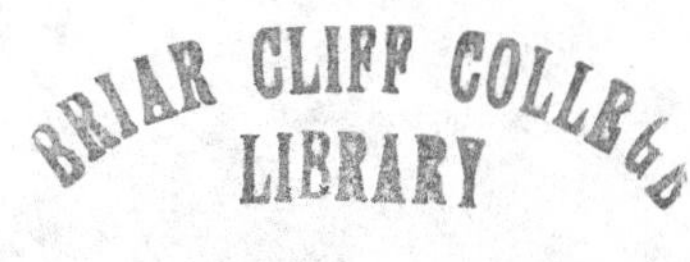

AN ASPEN PUBLICATION®
Aspen Systems Corporation
Rockville, Maryland
London
1982

Library of Congress Cataloging in Publication Data
Main entry under title:

Nursing education.

Includes bibliographical references and index.
1. Nursing—Study and teaching—Addresses, essays, lectures. I. Brown, Barbara J. II. Chinn, Peggy L., 1941-
RT71.N775 1982 610.73′07 82-11370
ISBN: 0-89443-807-7

Library of Congress Catalog Card Number: 82-11370
ISBN: 0-89443-807-7

Printed in the United States of America

1 2 3 4 5

Contents

Foreword

The problems found in nursing today are so complex that the National Commission on Nursing recognizes that no single proposed solution is possible. Nursing education and nursing service have continuously responded to issues with divergent points of view, fueling the growth of the schisms between practitioners and educators. Nursing education and nursing service together have been responsible for creating widespread misunderstanding about nursing. If the public is in a dilemma about how to respond to the nursing shortage, the need for nursing education funds, and the lack of role clarification in the nurse practitioner and other expanded role models, we have only the nursing profession itself to blame.

The selections in this volume focus on both the nursing education and nursing service points of view, and are intended to help nursing advance toward unification. It is doubtful that mismatches between nursing education supply and nursing service needs will ever be resolved. Resolutions begin to appear when educators and nursing service professionals address the barriers in the practice environment that interfere with "professional practice models." The supply of RNs is a continuous dilemma in many practice environments. Recruitment efforts portray, all too often, an inappropriate image of professional nursing, as evidenced in a recent issue of a major professional journal where a ballerina was featured as an advertising gimmick for professional nursing.

The shortage of nurses who wish to work in hospitals is in part due to maldistribution and lack of educational preparation for service needs. Maldistribution of nurses occurs in relation to educators' willingness to educate in the areas where the nurses are most needed. A recent private grant through a private university school of nursing focuses on rural nursing. We need more innovative programs to staff our rural and acute-shortage area nursing positions, in order to begin to respond to the maldistribution problem.

Another area of concern to nursing service is the lack of nurses who are willing to work nights and weekends. "In the old days," nurses were readily enculturated to the 24-hour, 7-day-a-week responsibility through clinical experiences designed to provide evening and night experiences. Today, students are given little or no experience with working evening or night shifts; yet this is the time when the highest level of independent decision making is required. It is no wonder that nurses are unwilling to work these hours. The educational experience does not prepare nurses for the reality of the service setting.

Another major barrier is the changing role of the RN in the practice arena. There is no differentiation between the knowledge and skill levels of associate-degree, diploma, baccalaureate or master's-degree graduates. There is little role identification to enable people in the service setting to clearly differentiate among the job descriptions for these individuals. Successful autonomy in nursing practice requires specific clinical knowledge and competency. The cliché of "they can analyze and synthesize but can't catheterize" is all too often true. Little information about the development of peer relationships between RNs, LPNs and non-RN staff is offered in curricula today. This impedes nurses' ability to adapt to the service setting. And certainly, the service setting has a responsibility to reeducate existing nurses to adapt to new ways. The relationship between education and service must be collaborative.

Many staff nurses do not accept the responsibility and accountability that professional nursing practice requires. Many nurses do not want to perform direct patient care activities, and RNs sometimes do not recognize the need for more RNs, and create unnecessary barriers for new graduates entering the system. Nurses have traditionally focused on responsibility to the hospital instead of to the patient, which is contrary to the philosophy and ethos of nursing education. We certainly need to look toward achieving uniform definitions of nursing in order to move forward with the changing role in nursing practice.

Collectively, we are wasting much nursing talent when we fractionalize practice environments by creating multiple therapy roles such as intravenous therapy and do not allow professional nurses of today to practice comprehensive, holistic nursing care. In order to facilitate the changing role of the RN, it is essential for the practice environment to redefine support systems for nursing. Therefore, another major barrier for nursing today is the organization's structure for practice. Documentation and charting methods need to be modified to coincide with the nursing process as it is taught in the present nursing educational system. Organizationally, nursing should be restructured to provide for shared decision making and increased participation by all staff. Too often, organizational settings provide subjective loyalties to long-term employees and impede the dynamic influence of creative ideas of more recent, professional nursing program graduates. It is imperative that nursing administrators recognize outmoded habits of thought regarding efficiency and cost effectiveness unless these thoughts also include the professional practice model. Efficiency and cost effectiveness do not preclude the practice of comprehensive, quality nursing care, as demonstrated in primary nursing.

Division of labor must focus on clinical decision-making activities to allow nurses to practice nursing in an unimpeded environment. This requires administrative leadership in dealing with the effect that these changes may have on other departments, for example, housekeeping, pharmacy, dietary and other disciplines such as social service, and occupational and physical therapy. It is imperative for nursing to redefine its support systems for nursing practice in order to encourage and nurture today's graduates. If job expectation is clearly defined based on educational preparation, the baccalaureate-entry-into-practice issue can lead to appropriate pay scales for increased responsibilities. In some practice environments, the change in standards of practice is rewarded with increments. For example, when the nurse passes a national certification examination in critical care, that nurse is increased one increment step in pay.

Our mutual support of the standards of practice, certification and credentialing in advancing nursing practice is imperative. We need to utilize RNs according to their levels of competency. Patient acuity indicators and patient categories are the best vehicles for clearly demonstrating that "a nurse is not a nurse is not a nurse." They make reimbursement for nursing, based on services rendered, possible.

Other areas of concern in the practice environment relate to outside influences on nursing. Faculties must respect the stressors in the practice environment and be able to address them objectively with multiple points of view. The outside influences in a practice environment should not be addressed from the self-serving perspective of nurses in nursing. These considerations are not limited to, but include, tenured positions and dealing with labor unions, strong negative reactions on the part of the community when nurses are picketing on the issues of comparable worth, organizational fit as a health care administrator and development of solidarity within nursing.

Nurse educators need to be better informed about the reimbursement systems controlled and monitored by state rate review commissions and third party payers. If each nurse practicing today had an understanding of the external considerations affecting the nursing practice environment, we would have a more unified approach to the nursing profession.

Another major focus in the professional practice environment is the preparation of nursing leaders. Some of the articles in this volume address the preparation of the nurse administrator. The field of nursing service administration is reaching a new interface in the total field of health care administration. Many programs focus on interdisciplinary health care administrative curriculum. We know we have a lack of nurse administrators with strategy planning capabilities; too many administrators have difficulties dealing with change and a strategic planning approach. Nurse leaders need skills in negotiating with boards of directors, boards of trustees, medical staffs and other departments.

We have a tendency to jump on band wagons without looking at how they will affect individual settings. Often there is a lack of long-range planning for change and too much emphasis on crisis nursing administration. Not only do we need strong education programs to support the role of a nurse administrator in finance, politics, interorganizational relationships and all the issues involved within the profession of nursing, but we also need to gird our strength by creating support systems to enable nurse executives to achieve an organizational fit in the practice environment.

We are only effective as leaders in the field of nursing service if our educational preparation addresses the reality of complex, multisystems of health care. An educational expansion into the areas of public relations, politics, economics and comprehensive understanding of the issues within nursing is essential if we are to blend education and service together in the practice environment.

—Barbara Brown, R.N., Ed.D., F.A.A.N.
July 1982

Preface

Since the founding of professional nursing by Florence Nightingale, the education of nurses has been through several evolutionary periods. Nightingale, who believed strongly that nursing requires a body of knowledge that is distinct from medical knowledge, advocated nursing education programs that were autonomous from physicians or hospitals. Many early schools of nursing established in America were founded on her model, but the forces of dominant hospital-related groups gradually eroded this model and most schools of nursing became apprenticeship programs under the direct control of hospital administrations. Leaders in nursing since the beginning of this century have recognized the need for nurses to be educated in academic programs where the humanities and liberal arts form a basis for advanced nursing education. By the mid-20th century, the profession was firmly committed to the need for baccalaureate and graduate education in nursing, and a major move began to end the apprenticeship type of learning of early hospital schools to academic programs in institutions of higher learning.

Today we are still faced with many major problems in nursing education, some of them growing directly out of the struggle to gain and retain control of nursing education by nurses. Many different groups in contemporary society have vested interests in the form and content of nursing education, including the public who receive nursing services; the administrators of hospitals and other agencies who hire nurse graduates, practicing registered nurses, physicians and other health care workers who work with nurses; and students who enter our programs. Each of these groups has somewhat different expectations of nursing education, but all share a common concern for the quality and effectiveness of nursing education programs.

The purpose of this volume is to present a compilation of articles from current nursing literature that addresses some of the problems of nursing education, views regarding the quality and effectiveness of programs in nursing, and research evidence that might assist in making decisions that effect nursing education programs. The collection is not comprehensive of all possible views regarding nursing education, nor does it provide easy answers to some of our difficult problems. It does, however, provide a reflection of some of the major current concerns that have appeared in recent literature and challenges further development in the field.

It is our hope that this volume will stimulate the reader to explore further some of the issues presented here, and to explore other concerns or problems that are not included here. The challenge for greater development of excellence in nursing education depends upon the members of the profession expressing a strong voice that can be heard by all concerned with the future of nursing.

—Peggy L. Chinn, R.N., Ph.D., F.A.A.N.
July 1982

CURRICULUM AND TEACHING APPROACHES

The Effects of Modularized Instruction and Traditional Teaching Techniques on Cognitive Learning and Affective Behaviors of Student Nurses

Loucine M.D. Huckabay, R.N., M.S., Ph.D., F.A.A.N.
Professor
Department of Nursing
California State University
Long Beach, California

As MORE STUDENTS enter schools of nursing, nursing faculty are faced with the problem of accommodating increasing numbers of students with diverse abilities and speeds of learning. Independent study (IS) and programmed instruction have provided two avenues for individualizing instruction. If one of the chief aims of education is to help the student develop the ability and desire for continued learning after formal education is completed, it seems essential to expose the student to such experiences and arrange the academic environment to encourage independent learning.

De Tornyay commented that such an experience for independent learning should enable the students to obtain information, formulate problems, find answers, and evaluate their progress. The instructor and the instructional materials can assist each student toward autonomy of action and thought. Nursing schools today have not effectively used the IS strategy to meet the increasing educational needs of the students.[1]

INDEPENDENT LEARNING SYSTEMS

Independent learning systems are designed to facilitate learning. Independent study implies that the area of learning is of specific concern to the learner. Methods of IS are based on the assumption that learning is an individual act or event that takes place entirely within the learner.[1-4]

Sorensen, in discussing the IS technique of the nursing honors program at the University of Arizona, pointed out that one of the major purposes of the program is to help students develop skill in IS and research by having them explore nursing problems and select one to investigate in depth through writing a thesis.[5] Although it is generally believed that the academically superior student benefits the most from the IS technique, this hypothesis has not been empirically tested.[1]

Tutorials are another type of IS used extensively in the English system of higher education. Clark applied this technique with undergraduate students in a zoology course in two American universities. The students attended classes and wrote one essay each week on the subject selected jointly by the student and the tutor. Reaction from students and tutors was favorable. However, the major criticism from the students was that they had insufficient time to prepare a weekly essay because of heavy course work in both this course and other college courses.[6]

Another extensive research project on IS was conducted by Antioch College.[3] This project included courses in humanities, social sciences, and sciences and had varied periods of IS. The researchers measured both cognitive and affective achievement and evaluated the effect of IS on "learning resourcefulness." The faculty recognized that not all students were ready to work independently and therefore provided training for independent work. Results of this experiment, although somewhat inconclusive, did show differences pertaining to subject matter.

MODULAR COURSES

Modular courses are a new form of IS. It is an innovative form of instruction that is in the process of being implemented in the California state universities and colleges. A learning module is a package containing the whole of instructional materials necessary for the learning of a subject matter.[7] Learning modules contain: 1. Behavioral objectives for the module; 2. Pretest; 3. Resource references (written materials, required readings from texts or journals); 4. Direction for learning experiences to achieve the module objectives (eg, active or passive performance activities, such as interviewing a patient, going to the laboratory, and practicing giving injections etc.); 5. Specification and direction for the use of audiovisual equipment necessary to achieve the objective; and 6. Posttest.

Modular courses have been described as "structured nonstructuring." Modules are "discrete units of study complete with performance objectives which establish guidelines for satisfactory student completion." A modular course is one "in which a number of these units are combined sequentially to provide an overview of a particular area of interest or a body of information."[8]

Modular courses can take a variety of

styles, forms, and lengths. They may deal with one specific area of a discipline or they may be interdisciplinary with a common theme. Most of them are self-paced, some require little or no formal instruction time, and others involve extensive interaction between student and instructor. Some modular courses are offered on a 3-, 6-, or 9-week basis; others are scheduled on quarter or semester bases with corresponding credit unit values.[4]

There are several modularized programs that have been initiated in the California state systems. California State University (CSU) at Fullerton offers an open module system of minicourses in the natural sciences; instructional media modules are being developed at CSU at Sacramento and at San Jose. None of these programs has been in nursing. Results of studies on the effectiveness of modular instruction to date have been contrary to expectations, although it must be emphasized that it is too early for any definitive evaluation.

Because independent study methods vary greatly in the amount of assistance given to students and in the patterning of structured instruction versus the independent learning periods, McKeachie suggested that excusing students from class attendance and giving them the freedom to structure their learning is one way to stimulate independent learning.[3] The results of such a procedure are not clear, but they do suggest that classroom experience is not essential for learning.

The strategy of IS in modular form enables students to be the masters of their environments, in charge of their learning, with the locus of control internalized. The relationship between locus of control (internal or external) and achievement motivation has been explored by numerous researchers and theoreticians.[9-12] These studies and many others have indicated a direct positive relationship between internal control and involvement in achievement-oriented activities. It may be that successful attempts in such activities reinforce an internal control orientation.

Based on Bloom's theory of mastery learning and its affective consequences and Gagne's theory of acquisition of knowledge, it is expected that students will learn the subject matter (cognitive behavior) and will have a positive feeling of achievement and mastery (affective behavior) as a result of modularized courses. These students can pace the rate of learning and feel that they have control over their learning, compared to those students who take the same course and content matter in a more structured traditional lecture-discussion method of instruction.[13-15]

LECTURE-DISCUSSION METHOD

The lecture-discussion method of instruction is one of the most common teaching strategies used in classroom teaching in colleges and nursing schools. Here the presentation is supplemented by audiovisual aids, and the students are encouraged to interrupt for questions, comments, and clarifications. McKeachie stated that the use of both lectures and discussion is a logical and popular choice in courses where the instructors wish not only to give information but also to develop concepts.[3]

The lecture can effectively (1) present new research findings that have not yet been published, (2) emphasize and clarify important meanings and thus channel the thinking of a group of students in the

The mixed method of instruction—module and lecture-discussion—provides students with advantages of both instructional techniques and counteracts their disadvantages.

given direction, (3) vitalize facts and ideas that may appear cold and lifeless on the printed pages of a book, (4) expose large groups of students to authorities to share firsthand experiences, and (5) convey the teachers' enthusiasm. Teachers' experience and special way of organizing materials presented with masterful delivery can also inspire their students.[1]

The disadvantages of the lecture method are (1) too much emphasis is placed on certain facts and materials and too little on the learning process, (2) the wants and desires of the teacher are emphasized to the exclusion of the student's needs, (3) dependence on the teacher as the final authority is fostered thus inhibiting exploratory learning behavior on the part of the students, (4) a passive type of learning that tends not to be retained is created in students, and (5) the locus of control is with the teacher rather than being shared with the students.[1]

A teaching strategy that simultaneously uses the mixed method of instruction—module and lecture-discussion—provides students with advantages of both instructional techniques and counteracts their disadvantages.

HYPOTHESES

Based on the previously established theoretical framework on motivation and locus of control, affective consequences of acquisition of knowledge, and research studies relevant to achievement motivation, the following hypotheses have been developed:

1. Students enrolled in the mixed method of instruction—module and lecture-discussion (MLD group)—will demonstrate significant increases in cognitive learning, when measured in terms of both objective and subjective tests, compared to those students enrolled in similar courses using either module alone (M group) or lecture-discussion (LD group) method of instruction.
2. Students enrolled in the M group will demonstrate significantly more cognitive learning, when measured in terms of both objective and subjective tests, than those students enrolled in the LD group.
3. The students enrolled in the MLD group will demonstrate affective behaviors significantly more than those enrolled in either the M group or the LD group.
4. Students enrolled in the M group will demonstrate affective behaviors significantly more than the LD group.

Operational definitions

Learning module: independent unit or package of instruction that contains all the necessary instructional materials for the learning of the subject matter and achievement of specific objectives.

Cognitive learning: amount of learning about the subject matter that has taken place in the learner, during 1 quarter, as a result of given instruction. It is measured by the difference in scores between pretest and posttest.

Affective behaviors: positive feelings expressed by the learner towards the course and the learning process as measured by the "affective measures" tool.

Module alone teaching strategy: teaching technique whereby the learner achieves the instructional objectives with limited or no guidance from the teacher.

Lecture-discussion teaching strategy: teaching technique whereby the teacher presents the content area relevant to the topic and objective at hand, using the format of the lecture and then opens the topic for further questions and discussion with the students in a formalized classroom setting.

Module with lecture-discussion teaching strategy: teaching technique whereby the teacher presents the content using the lecture format and opens the topic for further discussion questions and answers with the students. Students also use the independent learning modules in conjunction with the lecture and discussion.

METHOD

Design

The experimental design called for three groups of subjects tested both on pretests and posttests. The dependent variables were (1) cognitive learning (behavior) measured in terms of both objective tests and on subjective Likert type scale and (2) affective behavior. The independent variables were the different types of teaching strategy: (1) lecture-discussion (LD), (2) module (M), and (3) mixed module and lecture-discussion (MLD).

Subjects

The subjects (Ss) were the graduate nursing students enrolled in a nursing education course at a large university in Southern California (N = 97). Group 1 (LD group) had 32 Ss who were those students enrolled in first quarter. Group 2 (M group) had 40 Ss who were those students enrolled in the second quarter. Group 3 (MLD group) had 25 Ss who were those students enrolled in the third quarter. To avoid contamination between students, the groups were studied a year apart. Subjects in each group were equated (matched), by means of pretests, in terms of level of knowledge they possessed about principles of learning and instruction prior to instruction. The subjects were also matched in terms of grade point average (GPA), age, and marital status. For all Ss the GPA was 3.0 and above. The mean ages for groups 1, 2, and 3 were 29.6, 31.7, and 30.2, respectively. No other control measures were placed on selection of Ss.

Procedure

Each subject in each group took three tests, two cognitive and one affective. The cognitive tests (objective and subjective) were administered in pretests and posttests. The affective test was administered only at the end of the course. At the beginning of the course each student in the class was given the pretest (objective and subjective) and was asked to answer each of the questions. The posttest was given at the completion of instruction. The affective measure was given only on the last day of class, and students were asked to rate themselves on this scale.

The method of instruction was as follows: The course consisted of 30 subject areas (topics) taught over a 10-week period (1 quarter). The content dealt with conditions of learning and instruction in nursing. All three groups received the exact same content taught by the same teacher. For group 1 (LD group), the teacher lectured on each subject and opened the topic for further discussion during each class period. The classes and reading assignments were conducted in a usual manner.

For group 2 (M group), the conduct of classes was based on IS method. Each of the 30 subject areas (topics) was placed on a module. The modules were placed both in the library on 2-hour reserve and in the school's learning lab. The scheduled class hours were left open for individual counseling and instruction if needed. For group 3 (MLD group), the procedures for lecture and module system were combined. During the regular scheduled class hours, the teacher lectured and conducted the discussion. The students also used the modules that were available in the library.

Instruments

Cognitive measures I (objective test)

The purpose of this instrument is to tap the student's amount of knowledge acquisition as a result of different teaching strategies. It consists of two parts; each part has 80 objective questions ranging from "True" and "False" category to multiple choice questions to matching questions. Part I deals with the conditions of learning; part II deals with conditions of instruction and variables influencing both learning and instruction.

Because there are 80 questions in each part and there are two parts, each question is assigned a score of 0.625 points and the total score for this instrument could therefore range from 0 to 100. The amount of cognitive learning is then calculated by subtracting the pretest score from posttest score.

The content validity of this instrument is based on literature; most of the questions are derived from four textbooks as well as from lecture notes, modules, and other current research studies.[16-19] Validity measure is also obtained through a panel of five judges who were former graduate students enrolled in the same courses the previous quarter. All five judges agreed that the content of the test is covered in the specified nursing education course, and there was 100% agreement on this measure.

The reliability of this instrument was obtained by means of a test-retest method. Twenty students took the retest 3 weeks after first testing. The Spearman rank correlation between test-retest was .8697, $p < .01$.

Cognitive measures II (subjective measure)

The purpose of this instrument is to measure the degree to which the students subjectively estimate the amount of knowledge they have acquired from the given course taught in a given manner. The instrument consists of 15 questions. Each question taps the extent to which each student perceives accomplishment of the objectives of the course. The instrument is constructed on a Likert rating scale; the range is from 0, indicating no knowledge, to 10, indicating perfect knowledge. Because there are 15 questions, the score could then range from 0 to 150.

The content validity of this instrument is based on the literature.[14,16,17,19] Also, a panel of five judges who were former graduate students enrolled in the same course the previous quarter rated the instrument. There was 100% agreement on this instrument.

Reliability was obtained by means of a test-retest method. Twenty students took the retest three weeks after first testing. Spearman rank correlation between test-retest was .9435, $p < .001$.

Affective measures

The purpose of this instrument is to tap students' feelings about the course and its method of instruction. The rationale of this instrument is based upon Bloom's theory on mastery learning, that positive feelings about the course and about the learning process will initiate a sense of achievement in the students and desire for more learning.[14] The instrument consists of 10 questions constructed on a Likert-type scale, ranging from 0, indicating unfavorable responses, to 10, indicating favorable responses (feelings, opinions, etc.) about the method of instruction. The eleventh item on this instrument asks the students about their preferences on method of instruction. It was scored and analyzed separately. Because there are 10 questions in this instrument, each ranging from 0 to 10 score, the total score on this instrument could then range from 0 to 100.

The content validity of this instrument is based on the literature.[11,14] A panel of five judges who were former graduate students enrolled in the same course the previous quarters also rated the instrument. There was 93.2% agreement between the judges.

The reliability was obtained by means of the test-retest method. The Spearman rank correlation between test-retest was .6310, $p < 0.01$. Twenty students took the retest 3 weeks after initial testing.

Demographic data

In addition to the above three instruments, minimum demographic data were obtained to determine if the extraneous variables of age, educational background, and marital status affect the dependent variables.

Method of analysis

The hypotheses were tested by means of one-way analysis of variance and t-test to determine if there were significant mean differences between the groups on cognitive learning and affective behaviors.

McNemar's test for symmetry was conducted to determine if students preferred one method of instruction over another.

Pearson's product-moment correlation (r) was conducted to determine if the extraneous, the dependent, and the independent variables are related to each other.

RESULTS

The first hypothesis proposed that students enrolled in group 3, which used the teaching strategy of module with lecture-discussion (MLD), would demonstrate a more significant increase in cognitive learning when measured in terms of objective tests (ACLO) and subjective tests (ACLS) than those students who were

Table 1. Analysis of variance for cognitive learning when measured in terms of objective test (ACLO)

Variable	SS	DF	MS	*F*-ratio	Probability
Between groups	4658.72	2	2339.36	21.60	0.00001
Within groups	10137.86	94	107.85		
Total	14796.58	96			

SS = Sum of squares
DF = Degree of freedom
MS = Means square

enrolled in either the module (M) or the lecture-discussion (LD) group.

One-way analysis of variance indicated that there were significant differences between the groups on cognitive learning when measured in terms of objective tests ($F = 21.60$, $p < .00001$) (see Table 1) but not with subjective tests ($F = 1.56$, $p < .21$) (see Table 2) even though the trend observed was in the predicted direction.

With regard to the objective tests, to determine between which groups the differences were occurring, Duncan's new multiple range test (DNMRT) revealed that the significant differences were occurring between the MLD and LD group at the $p < .01$ level. The differences between the MLD and the M group were not significant even though the trend observed was in the predicted direction (see Table 3). Therefore, the first hypothesis is partially supported.

The second hypothesis proposed that the M group will demonstrate significantly more cognitive learning, when measured in terms of both objective and subjective tests, than the LD group. Results of the *t*-test presented in Table 4 show that the M group has learned significantly more than the LD group when measured in terms of objective test ($t = -5.11$, $p < .001$) but not significant when measured in terms of subjective tests, even though the trend observed was in the predicted direction (see Table 3). Therefore, the second hypothesis is partially supported.

Another very important finding was discovered when comparisons were made *within* each group by means of the *t* test. Results presented in Table 5 indicate that

Table 2. Analysis of variance for cognitive learning when measured in terms of subjective test (ACLS)

Variable	SS	DF	MS	*F*-ratio	Probability
Between groups	1204.52	2	602.26	1.5642	0.2147
Within groups	36193.45	94	385.04		
Total	37397.97	96			

SS = Sum of squares
DF = Degree of freedom
MS = Means square

Table 3. Means and standard deviation on major variables

Group	Pre-O	Pre-S	Post-O	Post-S	ACLO	ACLS	Affect
MLD							
Mean	43.77	24.04	97.10	130.08	53.33	106.04	86.12
S.D.	9.58	11.43	1.89	9.33	10.05	13.78	6.97
M							
Mean	43.17	21.15	92.61	123.55	49.44	102.40	68.72
S.D.	10.05	18.46	5.15	17.00	10.06	22.75	17.61
LD							
Mean	44.01	28.78	80.58	125.75	36.57	96.97	81.50
S.D.	9.87	17.85	7.86	10.52	11.02	19.22	9.20

MLD = Module with lecture-discussion group
M = Module group
LD = Lecture-discussion group
S.D. = Standard deviation
Pre-O = Pretest measured in terms of objective tests
Pre-S = Pretest measured in terms of subjective tests
Post-O = Posttest measured in terms of objective tests
Post-S = Posttest measured in terms of subjective tests
Affect = Affective behavior

irrespective of teaching strategy all groups had learned significantly. The differences between posttest scores and pretest scores measured both objectively and subjectively were significant.

The third hypothesis proposed that the MLD group will demonstrate significantly more affective behaviors than either the M group or the LD group. Results of a one-way analysis of variance presented in Table 6 show that there were significant differences between the groups on affective behaviors ($F = 16.12, p < .00001$), but DNMRT showed that the significant differences occurred only between the MLD and the M groups at the $p < .01$ level and not between MLD and LD groups, even though the trend observed was in the predicted direction. The third hypothesis is therefore partially supported.

Table 4. Comparison of mean differences between groups by means of *t*-test on amount of cognitive learning (ACLO, ACLS) and affective behaviors

Groups	ACLO	ACLS	Affective
LD vs M			
t-value	-5.11	-1.10	3.96
p-value	.0001	.276	.0001

Results indicate that irrespective of teaching strategy all groups had learned significantly.

The fourth hypothesis proposed that the M group would demonstrate significantly more affective behaviors than the LD group. Results of the *t* test presented in Tables 3 and 4 show that the reverse is true: the LD group demonstrated signifi-

Table 5. Comparison of mean differences within groups by means of *t*-test

Group	ACLO (Post-O)-(Pre-O)	ACLS (Post-S)-(Pre-S)
LD		
t-value	18.77	28.55
p-value	0.00001	0.00001
M		
t-value	31.07	28.46
p-value	0.00001	0.00001
MLD		
t-value	26.54	38.49
p-value	0.00001	0.00001

cantly more affective behaviors than the M group ($t = 3.96, p < .0001$).

Additional findings

There were no significant differences between the groups on any of the extraneous variables of age, marital status, and educational background (ladder B.S. vs. generic B.S.) when tested in terms of the chi-square test. Correlational tests also showed no significant relationships between the extraneous variable of age and the dependent variables.

To determine if students preferred one teaching strategy over another and if there were changes from the strategy they received to what they preferred, McNemar's test for symmetry (McTs) was performed. Results presented in Table 7 indicate that there were significant changes from the teaching strategy they had to what they preferred. Students preferred the MLD strategy significantly more than the other teaching techniques (McTs value = 46.091, $p < .01$).

To compare if the students' subjective evaluations of their level of knowledge are similar to those measured by means of objective tests and if they are related to one another, a *t* test and Pearson's product moment correlations (r) were performed. Results of the *t* test, presented in Table 8, show significant differences between objective test and subjective test (self-evaluation). The *t* test value for the pretest ($t = 19.19, p < .00001$) and posttest ($t = 4.71, p < .001$) indicate that subjective test scores were significantly lower than objective test scores. But for amount of cognitive learning (ALCO, ACLS) ($t = -13.96,$

Table 6. Analyses of variance for affective behavior

Variable	SS	DF	MS	*F*-ratio	Probability
Between groups	5449.08	2	2724.54	16.12	0.00001
Within groups	15890.59	94	169.05		
Total	21339.67	96			

Table 7. McNemar's Test for symmetry for changes from strategy received to strategy preferred

Strategy Preferred	Strategy Received LD	M	MLD	Total
LD	6	2	0	8
M	2	8	3	13
MLD	24	30	22	76
Total	32	40	25	97

McNemar's Test for Symmetry Value = 46.091 (obtained)
$df = 3$
$p < .00001$
LD = Lecture discussion
M = Module
MLD = Module with lecture discussion

$p < .00001$), the subjective testing was higher than objective evaluations.

Correlations

The correlation matrix shows that pretest scores measured both objectively (Pre-O) and subjectively (Pre-S) are related to one another positively but not significantly. Similarly, the posttest scores measured objectively (Post-O) and subjectively (Post-S) are positively related to one another but not significantly. However, the amounts of cognitive learning measured objectively (ACLO) and subjectively (ACLS) are positively and significantly related to one another ($r = .2976, p < .01$).

Table 8. Comparison of mean differences between objective and subjective evaluation by means of *t*-test on major variables

Group	Pretest	Post-test	ACL
Obj vs. *subj*			
t-value	19.19	4.71	-13.96
p-value	0.00001	0.0001	0.01

ACL = Amount of cognitive learning = Posttest-pretest
obj = objective testing
subj = subjective testing

Other significant correlational findings are: (1) the Pre-O scores are inversely and significantly correlated with ACLO ($r = -.7109, p < .001$); (2) the Pre-S scores are inversely and significantly correlated with ACLO ($r = -.2298$, $p < .05$), with ACLS ($r = -.7393$, $p < .0001$) and with Post-O ($r = -1960, p < .05$); (3) the Post-O scores are positively and significantly correlated with both ACLO ($r = .6221, p < .001$) and with ACLS ($r = .2077$, $p < .05$); (4) the Post-S scores are positively and significantly correlated with ACLS ($r = .5384$, $p < .01$); and (5) the affective behaviors are positively and significantly correlated with Post-S scores ($r = .4949$, $p < .01$) and ACLS ($r = .2146, p < .05$).

DISCUSSION

The significant positive findings on the first hypothesis indicate that students enrolled in a class where the MLD method of instruction was implemented did acquire significantly more cognitive knowledge than the LD group when measured in terms of objective tests (ACLO) but not when measured by means of subjective tests, even though the trend observed in the latter situation was in the direction of prediction. The significant finding is consistent with the theoretical framework of achievement motivation that proposes that when the locus of control to master a task or one's own environment is internal, the individual tends to get involved in achievement oriented activities.[9-12]

Findings are also consistent with Rotter's view of achievement motivation that proposes that motivation to achieve a specific goal is a function of the expectation an individual has for reaching the goal and the value placed on the outcome.[13] The teaching strategy of MLD that was implemented with the third group provided students with the control to master the learning task because within this strategy students could pace their learning and study content areas as many times as they felt were necessary to master the subject matter. The students also had the freedom not to attend the class sessions if they so desired, but almost all the students enrolled in this class attended the class sessions approximately 90% of the time.

Explicit goals

The modular course with LD that was implemented with the MLD group makes the goals and objectives of the learning task explicit and arranges these tasks from the simple to the complex so that students undertake the task when they are ready and have mastered all the prerequisite subordinate tasks. Furthermore, the fact that this course was an elective and not a required course for graduation indicates that students value the outcome of the course.

Lack of significant differences between the MLD and M group can be explained by the fact that the teaching strategy of module alone (M) is an independent study. It also provides students with a locus of control that is internal because they can pace their own learning and it also makes the expectation of the course explicit. Students also value the outcome of the course. Apparently not having the additional positive assets of the LD strategy did not make a significant difference in cognitive learning between the MLD and the M group. It seems that the teaching strategy of M alone is adequate to achieve the course objectives. The fact that the MLD group had the additional positive asset of having the teacher lecture about the content and open the topics for discussion did produce more learning in the MLD group but not significantly more than the M group.

Objective and subjective measurements

Lack of significant differences between the groups on cognitive learning when measured in terms of subjective tests may be due to the fact that subjective evaluations are not as accurate as the objective methods of evaluations. The subjective and objective test scores on the posttest were not significantly correlated with one another. These findings are consistent with the recent study of Huckabay and Arndt in which they found that in general students tend to overestimate or underestimate the level of knowledge they possess about a topic at a given point in time.[20] The only finding that was significantly correlated was the amount of knowledge they had acquired when measured in terms of objective (ACLO) and subjective (ACLS) tests. The latter findings can be explained from Bloom's point of view that when learners accomplish or master the subject matter (task), they experience subjective feelings of achievement and success.[14]

The second hypothesis proposed that the M group would demonstrated significantly more cognitive learning when measured in terms of both objective and subjective tests than the LD group. The hypothesis is fully supported when objective tests are used but not when subjective tests are used, even though in the latter situation the trend is in the predicted direction. The significant findings are again consistent with theories of achievement motivation that propose that achievement activities such as mastering a task is a function of having a locus of control that is internal, making goals in the form of expectations explicit and attainable, and placing value on the outcome of the task. The teaching strategy of module alone in the form of independent study meets these criteria.[9-13]

Lack of strong support for this hypothesis when measured in terms of objective tests may be accounted for by the nature of the subjective tests. As mentioned previously, findings of both this study as well as Huckabay and Arndt's study point out that subjective tests do not provide an accurate method of evaluating learning.[20] Students tended to either overestimate or underestimate the level of cognitive knowledge they possess.

Another interesting finding was discovered when comparisons were made *within* each group. Irrespective of the teaching strategy, there were significant differences between pretest and posttest scores on cognitive learning when measured both objectively and subjectively, indicating that all subjects had learned significantly. These findings are consistent in part with theories of achievement motivation and also with Gagne's theory of acquisition of knowledge, which states that attainment of a new learning set is dependent upon recall of relevant subordinate learning sets and effect of instruction.[15] In this study, students apparently made use of their previously learned learning sets (basic knowledge in theories of learning and instruction) and built upon them the new learning sets of higher order principles of learning and instruction. Even though the effect of instruction did make a difference between the groups, it also provided the students enrolled in different strategies with learning experiences that were appropriate in achieving course objectives and produce significant learning.

Affective behavior differences

The third hypothesis, which proposed that the MLD group would demonstrate significantly more affective behaviors than either the M group or the LD group, was supported when comparisons were made between MLD and M group but not between the MLD and LD groups, even though in the latter situation the trend observed was in the predicted direction. The significant finding is consistent with Bloom's and Block's theory on mastery learning that advocates that positive feelings (affective behaviors) about the course and the content area and the desire for more learning (intrinsic motivation) are generated when students perceive and experience success and feel important.[14,17]

This is also substantiated by the significant correlational finding between affective behavior and amount of cognitive knowledge (ACLO, ACLS) that was acquired. (See Table 9.) The fact that the MLD group experienced more affective

Table 9. Correlation matrix for major variables

Variable	Pre-O	Post-O	Pre-S	Post-S	ACLO	ACLS	Affective	Age
Pre-O	1							
Post-O	.1084	1						
Pre-S	.1154	-.1960*	1					
Post-S	-.1351	.0587	.1694	1				
ACLO	-.7109‡	.6221‡	-.2298*	.1480	1			
ACLS	-.1913	.2077*	-.7393‡	.5384†	.2976†	1		
Affective	.0816	-.0546	.1445	.4949†	-.1029	.2146*	1	
Age	-.1337	-.0842	.1442	-.0065	-.0457	-.1277	-.0558	1

*$p < .05$
†$p < .01$
‡$p < .001$
Pre-O = Pretest measured by means of objective test
Pre-S = Pretest measured by means of subjective test
Post-O = Posttest measured by means of objective tests
Post-S = Posttest measured by means of subjective tests
ACLO = Amount of cognitive learning measured by means of objective test
ACLS = Amount of cognitive learning measured by means of subjective test

behaviors than the M group even though both groups had learned equally well can be explained by de Tornyay's view of the affective aspects of lecture-discussion teaching strategy utilizing a live teacher.[1] Since the MLD group was exposed to a live teacher who lectured and discussed each topic with the students, this strategy may have provided the students with a subject matter that was more vital than might have otherwise appeared on a printed page. Furthermore, the LD strategy may have conveyed the teacher's enthusiasm. Her experience and special way of organizing materials presented with masterful delivery may have also served as a motivating and inspiring experience for her students.

The lack of significant difference in affective behavior between the MLD and LD group may also be accounted for by these affective consequences of the LD method of instruction because the students enrolled in LD teaching strategy were exposed to the same teacher who implemented the same type of LD teaching technique. As shown in Table 5, these students had also acquired a significant amount of cognitive knowledge and had accomplished the course objectives satisfactorily, even though their learning was not as great as that of the students enrolled in MLD group. Therefore the fact that the LD group had accomplished the course objectives satisfactorily and had personal contact with the teacher within the LD strategy was enough to give them affective feelings of satisfaction and achievement.

The fourth hypothesis proposed that the M group would demonstrate significantly higher effective behaviors than the LD group. The reverse of this hypothesis was supported. The fact that the M group not only did not demonstrate significantly more affective behavior than the LD group, but less, may indicate that acquisition of knowledge *alone* is not sufficient to create or initiate intrinsic motivation in the form of desire for more learning, or its worthwhileness.

One additional observation was made by the teacher that is worth reporting: approximately one-sixth of the M class dropped out of the course at the end of the first week of instruction. Some of the reasons given were: "I miss not seeing the teacher," "I miss the teacher contact," "I want to hear the teacher's point of view," "I heard that the teacher was a dynamic lecturer; I miss not having that," "I was missing something," and other points to the same effect.

The superior affective behavior of the LD group can again be accounted for in terms of the role of the affective consequences of the LD teaching strategy as pointed out by de Tornyay and by the fact that they had acquired a significant amount of knowledge to accomplish the course objectives satisfactorily even though it was not as much as M group.[1]

Findings on the choice of teaching strategy indicate that learners overwhelmingly preferred the MLD over the M alone or the LD alone teaching strategies. This may indicate that students prefer a teaching strategy that has a two-way communication process between themselves and the teacher and want to pace their own learning and feel that they have control over the learning environment and the task.

Findings on the other correlational data follow a logical order with a common sense explanation. The significant inverse correlation between pretest scores (Pre-O, Pre-S) and amount of cognitive learning (ACLO, ACLS) can be explained by the fact that the less students know at the beginning of the course, the more they will learn by the completion of instruction. This finding is also consistent with Huckabay and Arndt's study.[20] The significant positive correlation between posttest scores (Post-O, Post-S) and amount of cognitive learning (ACLO, ACLS) can be explained by the fact that posttest scores determine the level of knowledge students have acquired at the completion of instruction. Amount of cognitive learning (ACL) indicates how much they have learned. ACL is determined by subtracting pretest scores from posttest scores.

The findings of this study have many implications for the education of nursing students and for inservice education.

APPLICATIONS OF RESULTS

The findings of this study have many implications for the education of nursing students and for inservice education. For example, if one of the objectives of the teacher or the nurse is to enable the student or the staff member to acquire knowledge about a content area such as diet, disease conditions procedures, type of care, and so forth, then the implementation of a teaching strategy that utilizes independent learning modules with lecture-discussion will produce in general the most amount of learning in students or staff than either the module alone or only the traditional LD teaching method.

It is also important to stress that if the teacher or the nurse does not have access to an independent learning module but has access to a good lecturer, or does not have a knowledgeable person to lecture and discuss a specific topic but has access to a learning module, the implementation of either M alone or LD alone will produce significant learning in the students or staff.

The findings of this study can also be used by the nurse teacher to reduce the teacher-student ratio. For example, teachers with a large number of students can divide the group into smaller groups. While one group is studying with the use of the modules, the teacher can meet with the other group and lecture on the topic and then open the subject area for discussion. Then the groups can exchange places. Reduced teacher-student ratios enhance more student participation and more individualization. Also, studying with the use of the modules enables students to pace their own learning according to their individual needs. Therefore it is also a method of handling individual differences in learning.

The third major and very important educational implementation of this study is in the area of affective learning in the forms of generating intrinsic motivation for more learning, taking initiative for one's own learning, and liking what one is learning. If one of the main aims of nursing education and practice is to enable the student or the staff nurse to continue learning after formal education or learning sessions are over, then the utilization of the MLD teaching method and the opportunity for the teacher to have personal contact with the learner should be provided during the teaching-learning process.

Limitations of the study

Even though the subjects in each of the groups were matched with respect to entering behavior on content taught, age, marital status, and grade point average, their level of motivation, cognitive style, and the interaction effect between student characteristics and teaching strategy were not controlled. It would have been more desirable to have had subjects assigned randomly to each of the groups. However, under the naturalistic setting of this educational environment, this was not possible.

Suggestions for further research

It is recommended that this study be replicated using a larger sample and under more controlled conditions, and that study be extended to answer the following questions:

1. Should the LD precede or follow the independent learning module to produce the most amount of cognitive and affective learning in learners?
2. Does the teaching strategy of independent learning module accompanied by LD that is given by a *live* teacher versus an MLD strategy with a *videotaped* (film) lecturer produce the same amount of cognitive and affective learning in students?

REFERENCES

1. de Tornyay R: *Strategies for Teaching Nursing.* New York, John Wiley & Sons, 1971.
2. Gagne RM: *Learning and Individual Differences.* Columbus, Ohio, Charles Merrill Books, 1967.
3. McKeachie WJ: Procedures and techniques of teaching: a survey of experimental studies, in Sanford, N (ed): *The American College.* New York, John Wiley & Sons, 1966.
4. Bevis EO, Bower F: *A workshop in individualized learning modalities.* Unpublished manuscript distributed at workshop at the University of California, San Francisco School of Nursing, March 27-28, 1973.
5. Sorensen G: An honors program in nursing. *Nurs Outlook* 16:59-61, 1968.
6. Clark RB: An experiment with tutorials, *J Higher Educ* 26:195-199, 1955.
7. Bevis EO: *Curriculum Building in Nursing: A Process.* St. Louis, The CV Mosby Co, 1973.
8. Future Talk. *Chancellors Newsletter,* no. 2 Sacramento, California State University Colleges.
9. Allport GW: *Becoming.* New Haven, Conn, Yale University Press, 1955.
10. Coleman J et al: *Equality of Educational Opportunity, Final Report.* US Report No. 38001. US National Center for Educational Statistics, 1966.
11. Crandall VC, Katkovsky W, Crandall VJ: Children's belief in their control of reinforcement in intellectual-academic achievement situations. *Child Devel* 36:91-109, 1965.
12. Wolk S, DuCette J. The moderating effect of locus of control in relation to achievement-motivation variables. *J Personal* 41:59-70, 1973.
13. Rotter JB: Generalized expectancies for internal vs. external control of reinforcement. *Psychol Monog* 80:1, 1966.
14. Bloom BS: Affective consequences of school achievement, in Block JH (ed) *Mastery Learning: Theory & Practice.* New York, Holt, Rinehart and Winston, 1971, pp 13-28.
15. Gagne RM. The acquisition of knowledge. *Psychol Rev* 69:355-365, 1962.
16. DeCecco J, Crawford W: *The Psychology of Learning and Instruction: Educational Psychology,* ed 2. Englewood Cliffs, NJ, Prentice-Hall, 1975.
17. Block JH: *Mastery Learning: Theory & Practice.* New York, Holt, Rinehart and Winston, 1970.
18. Gagne RM: *The Conditions of Learning,* ed 2. New York, Holt, Rinehart and Winston, 1970.
19. Ellis H: *The Transfer of Learning.* New York, The MacMillan Co, 1965.
20. Huckaby LM: D, Arndt C: The effect of acquisition of knowledge on self-evaluation and the relationship of self-evaluation to perception of real and ideal self-concept. *Nurs Res* 25:244-251, 1976.

The Relationship Between Senior Nursing Students' Ability to Formulate Nursing Diagnoses and the Curriculum Model

Vivien DeBack, R.N., M.S., Ph.D.
Associate Professor
Chairperson
Division of Nursing
Alverno College
Milwaukee, Wisconsin

BACCALAUREATE NURSING EDUCATION proposes to prepare the graduate in the use of the nursing process, which is the problem-solving methodology distinctive to professional nursing practice. Formulation of nursing diagnoses as a part of the nursing process is an assumed outcome of this educational preparation. Although problem solving in nursing is a skill taught in the baccalaureate curriculum, the nursing theories on which various curricula are based differ.

Nursing educators who subscribe to a variety of nursing theories frequently apply an eclectic approach to curriculum development. This combination of various theoretical formulations intrinsic to the science of nursing results in nursing curricula decidedly different in curriculum objectives although sharing common goals of nursing education. Therefore in this study the curriculum models of baccalaureate schools of nursing have been categorized to relate curriculum categories to the diagnostic abilities of senior nursing students. Secondary questions of relationships between ability to formulate nursing diagnoses and teaching strategies and assessment methods are also addressed in this research.

RATIONALE FOR THE STUDY

Nursing education has been examined throughout the twentieth century, beginning in 1923 with the Goldmark study.[1] Since then there have been continual efforts to restructure nursing educational institutions and curricula.

A review of nursing curricula over time indicates that a variety of curriculum designs have been developed. Within these designs are common goals of nursing education, such as "to promote the health of individuals and society." Professional goals of this kind are reflected in the outcomes in specific schools that are as varied as the faculty that staff them. Curriculum outcomes in baccalaureate nursing education are developed based on a particular theoretical approach to the scientific discipline of nursing. Although there are several theoretical approaches, the outcomes of each school specify what the faculty believe the practice of nursing to be. Thus these curriculum outcomes define the person who receives nursing care, the purpose of nursing, and the activities that the nurse performs.

Theoretical constructs in nursing have been identified by several nurse theorists, and curriculum models have been developed to facilitate thinking about concepts and the relationships among them. Several curriculum models for baccalaureate education have been developed, and the curricula that emerge from them do differ from each other. Thus any study of nursing education will of necessity require categorizing curricula of schools of nursing according to their curriculum model. Baccalaureate schools categorized according to curriculum model constitute the major independent variable for this study In this study curriculum models include the organization of content as well as the approach to the client.

Although educators in baccalaureate nursing programs subscribe to common professional goals and develop diverse curricula based on those goals, the nursing profession has identified the nursing process as a specific activity that distinguishes it from other health care disciplines. This problem-solving method is taught by educators in baccalaureate schools of nursing.

The nursing process includes five distinct types of activity: assessment (data collection), nursing diagnosis (problem identification), plan (goals), interventions (actions of the nurse), and evaluation. The nursing diagnosis step in the process requires a high level of intellectual skill and is a crucial ability in nursing activities. This step is the most strategic aspect of the process and concludes the assessment component. In the absence of a problem identification there is no need to continue with the other components of the process because there would exist no objective basis for planning, for intervention, or for evaluative judgments about the client's problems.[2]

Diagnostic ability of senior nursing students was the focus of this study. To evaluate this ability, nursing care plans of senior nursing students in baccalaureate schools were analyzed. The analysis consisted of applying predetermined criteria to the nursing diagnosis step of the nursing process that had been recorded by a student on a nursing care plan.

The student's ability to formulate nursing diagnoses was then related to the type of curriculum model selected by the faculty of the school to determine the relative relationship of ability and curriculum model.

LITERATURE REVIEW

Although evaluation of student achievement is a universal and frequent occurrence in baccalaureate programs, there is considerable difficulty obtaining data on student achievement at campus level. Studies exist that provide information on how colleges have influenced the attitudes, beliefs, and characteristics of students, but there is little information about students' acquisition of specific knowledge and skills.[3]

Evaluation of problem solving as a generic ability has not been a subject of extensive research. At the college level, the skill of problem solving is commonly integrated with the knowledge component of a discipline. Most studies of student achievement specify attainment of knowledge of the subject rather than the process ability of problem solving within the context of the discipline.

In recent years problem-solving ability has been identified as a generic competence in the core curriculum of College IV at Grand Valley State College in Michigan and at Alverno College in Milwaukee, Wisconsin.[4,5] Although programs of studies in other colleges and universities claim problem solving as an outcome, the methods for achieving that skill are not as explicitly defined as at College IV and Alverno.

Although studies documenting the problem-solving ability of college students or the relationship of that ability to the college experience are scarce, evidence related to what happens between the time students enter and leave an institution of higher education is equally scarce. However, the available evidence is generally consistent. Students change during the college years, and the intellectual status of college graduates is demonstrably different from that of nongraduates.[6]

In the nursing literature there is little evidence of evaluation or comparison of outcomes of baccalaureate education. This may be partly due to the fact that the curricula developed for nursing education differ, resulting in lack of comparative data. However, it would seem that even though the specific courses preparing the graduate nurse are diverse, some outcomes should be similar. It also seems likely that these similarities could be assessed in students from different schools.

Matthews and Gaul[7,8] conducted two studies to determine the specific variables that relate to nurses' cognitive abilities to process information during the nursing diagnostic process. Significant correlations were found in undergraduates in the concept attainment study[7] between the scores on the Concept Mastery Test and the cue perception in the diagnosis of impaired elimination. In the critical thinking study[8] there was no significant difference between the graduates' and undergraduates' abilities to engage in critical thinking as measured by the Watson-Glaser Critical Thinking Appraisal. Based on the data from these two studies it was concluded that there was a difference between the undergraduate and graduate subjects in their ability to derive nursing diagnosis as determined in the Critical Thinking Study. However, there was no overall relationship between the ability to derive nursing diagnoses and to think critically.

Little research exists, such as that of Gaul and Matthews, in which the thinking processes necessary for formulating nursing diagnoses have been studied. The literature review indicates a lack of research on the concept of nursing diagnoses, specifically the degree to which nurses are educated to formulate nursing diagnoses.

HYPOTHESES

The major hypothesis tested was that curriculum models will predict the relative ability of senior nursing students to formulate nursing diagnoses. Specifically, systems model curricula will predict greater ability in diagnoses formulation than other curriculum models.

Curriculum design is defined for this study as a term that includes the total instructional organization, curriculum model, teaching strategies, and assessment. Because of the close relationship of these variables to outcomes of education, two secondary hypotheses were developed. They are that (1) employment of student-involved teaching strategies will be associated with a greater ability to formulate nursing diagnoses by senior nursing students, and (2) employment of essay-type assessment methods rather than objective-type methods will be associated with greater ability to formulate nursing diagnoses by senior nursing students.

PHASE I

The purpose of Phase I of the study was to categorize baccalaureate schools of nursing according to the nursing theories that form the basis for their curricula.

Definitions of types of curriculum models were developed from the professional literature. Nursing theories having common elements were clustered under one model. This categorization reflected a composite of program foci and resulted in four curriculum groupings labeled models. These models were identified as developmental, systems, interaction, and medical.[9] (See boxed material.)

Based on the definitions of the models a questionnaire was developed. This instrument was composed of 24 statements, 6 of which described one of the four curriculum categories and were presented in scrambled order. The statements, developed from the model definitions, describe the function of the nurse, the goal of nursing, the major method of data collection used by students, the program organization, the content focus, and the client need. Items were not mutually exclusive. This allowed any school that teaches a combination of nursing theories to describe its curriculum by identifying all items that reflect that school's program.

The questionnaire was mailed to the deans of all baccalaureate nursing schools accredited by the National League for Nursing. Deans were asked to attempt to reflect their faculty's view rather than their own when responding to the instrument.

DEFINITIONS OF CURRICULUM MODELS

Medical model. A curriculum that is organized around disease processes. In this model the nursing role is directed toward alleviating the client problems resulting from a pathological condition. The curriculum focus is on symptoms and treatment as they are related to the medical regimen. Collection of data for the nursing process is guided by pathophysiological theories and health status alterations.

Interaction model.[10-12] A nursing curriculum that is organized around the understanding of human interpersonal relationships, particularly the individuals' perceptions of their status. The client's experience of health status is the key element in data collecting. In this model the nurse assists the client to avoid or alleviate the distress of unmet needs. To do so the nurse attempts to understand experiences that distress the client. This is accomplished through validation by the nurse of the client's perception of needs. The nursing goal is effective nurse interaction. Such interaction is directed toward learning the meaning, to a patient, of a particular experience. Collection of data about the nursing process is accomplished through direct observation by the nurse of the nurse-client interactions.

Developmental model.[13,14] A nursing curriculum that is organized around the concepts of fundamental human needs. Generally the theory basis is derived from the conceptualizations of Maslow and Erickson that postulate that each stage of life has specific goals or levels to be achieved and that change takes place from one level to another. In this model the nurse complements the client's ability by supplying what is needed in knowledge, will, or strength to perform daily activities. The curriculum focus is nursing assessment of basic human needs and the recognition of the individual's ability to grow and change in relation to those needs. Collection of data is guided by concepts underlying developmental theories.

Systems model.[15-17] A nursing curriculum that is organized around the stability or adaptation of the client. In this model the nurse's role is to assist the client to remain in or return to an adaptive state. The curriculum focus is total client care through assessment of the entire person and the person's relationship to the environment. The collection of data is accomplished through a systems approach in which the nurse analyzes each system for the purpose of manipulating the relationships, which may result in increased stability. The systems used are specified by each theorist, as for example, physiological, psychological, or environmental.

Additional data collected in Phase I on all schools of nursing included size of student body, geographic location, and public or private auspices.

PHASE II

The purpose of Phase II of the study was to determine the ability of senior nursing students to formulate nursing diagnoses and to relate that ability to the curriculum model. To achieve this objective, five schools were randomly selected from each of four curriculum categories. A further randomized selection was accomplished in each school by applying random numbers to an alphabetical list of senior students. Ten students in each school, selected in this manner, provided nursing care plans for analysis. The resultant pool of care plans (200) selected by this randomized method ensured the generalizability of the findings.

The basic design of the study called for a selection of five schools in each curricular category. After analyzing the data from Phase I, selection of schools in the medical model was not possible because no baccalaureate schools of nursing were categorized as medical model. However, 24% of the respondents received scores on the questionnaire that reflected a mixed curriculum category. Therefore five schools from this group were selected based on relatively high medical model scores.

A student response form was developed to help answer the two secondary hypotheses. This form fulfilled two purposes. First, answering the form constituted agreement on the part of the students to participate in the study, assured anonymity, and granted permission to have one of their nursing care plans analyzed with respect to the student's ability to formulate a nursing diagnosis. Secondly, the form was used to collect data about the major teaching strategies and assessment methods used in each school.

Analysis of the nursing care plans focused on the nursing diagnosis step of the nursing process. Specific criteria were used to determine the relative ability of senior nursing students to formulate a nursing diagnosis. Criteria were derived from the definition of nursing diagnosis developed by the participants in the National Conference on the Classification of Nursing Diagnosis.[18]

Analysis of the nursing care plans focused on the nursing diagnosis step of the nursing process.

The criteria as applied to a given diagnosis are: (1) Client rather than disease centered; (2) Stated in terms of client concerns and levels of competence or dysfunction; and (3) Statements of client concerns, competence, or dysfunction that can be altered or maintained through nursing action. Nursing care plans were scored according to both the total number of criteria and the specific criteria met. The method of scoring identified not only the number of criteria met but which criteria were met: none, criterion 1, criterion 2, or criterion 3. The purpose of this method of scoring was to determine the areas of strengths and deficits in the students' formulation of nursing diagnoses.

FINDINGS OF PHASE I

There were 417 questionnaires mailed during January 1980, and 270 (71%) were returned.

None of the 270 respondent schools could be categorized as a medical model based on the instrument used in this study. All of the 270 schools that returned the completed survey tool were categorized as representing one or more nursing models. The frequency distribution for each of the four curriculum categories and a fifth category labeled "mixed" is shown in Figure 1. Auspices (private or public) of the responding schools are also included.

Of the respondent schools in Phase I, 50% were categorized as systems model; 19% were categorized as developmental;

and 6% were interaction model. Respondent schools whose scores indicated that their curricula reflected beliefs and concepts common to more than one category identified in this study were categorized as having mixed models and totaled 24% of the sample.

Each nursing model in this study incorporates several nursing theories; therefore these data allow the conclusion that curricula in baccalaureate schools of nursing reflect an eclectic approach to curriculum design rather than a singular approach advanced by a single theorist.

Of the 270 respondent schools, 126 were private and 144 were public institutions. Nursing curricula identified in this study as developmental and systems models characterized 73% of the private schools in the sample. Of the schools categorized as

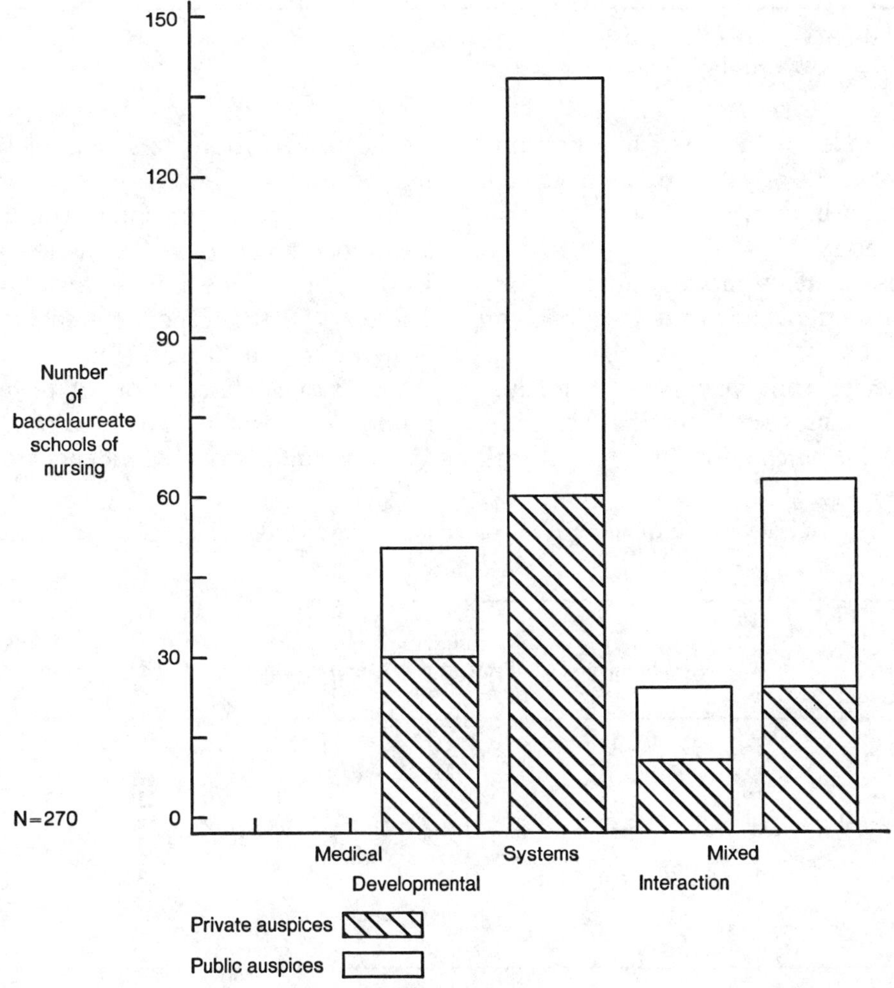

Fig 1. Frequency distribution of responses to phase I questionnaire: Baccalaureate schools of nursing categorized according to curriculum model and auspices.

Table 1. Baccalaureate schools of nursing categorized according to enrollment and curriculum model

		Curriculum model*								Schools not responding	
		Developmental		Systems		Interaction		Mixed			
Enrollment	N	*f*	%	*f*	%	*f*	%	*f*	%	*f*	%
901–999	2	0		1	50	0		0		1	50
751–500	14	0		10	71	0		0		4	29
601–750	16	1	6	6	38	1	6	5	31	3	19
451–600	25	4	17	10	43	0		5	16	6	24
301–450	71	6	8	26	37	1	1	9	13	29	41
151–300	127	17	13	43	34	6	5	28	22	33	26
30–150	127	23	18	39	31	10	8	19	15	36	28
Total	382**	51		135		18		66		112	

*No schools were classified as medical model.

**Of the 417 schools, 35 returned unanswered questionnaires.

systems model, 52% are public institutions. The most frequently occurring curriculum emphasis in both types of schools is the systems model.

Because systems model curricula were found more frequently in both public and private schools, it can be concluded that the perceived shift in nursing curriculum models, as suggested by the literature, from disease orientation (medical model) to client orientation (nursing model) has in fact occurred.

Developmental and interaction models are more frequently found in schools whose populations are less than 300. (See Table 1.) Of the respondent schools, 69% have fewer than 300 students.

Geographic distribution of respondent schools is shown in Table 2. Although the smallest number of respondents are found

Table 2. Baccalaureate schools of nursing categorized according to geographic region and curriculum model

		Curriculum model*								Schools not responding	
		Developmental		Systems		Interaction		Mixed			
Region	N	*f*	%	*f*	%	*f*	%	*f*	%	*f*	%
Northeast	79	10	13	32	41	5	6	12	15	20	25
Southeast	50	1	2	13	26	0		11	22	25	50
North central	73	18	25	33	45	5	6.8	10	13.6	7	9.6
South central	69	6	9	21	30.4	3	4.3	12	17.3	27	39
Midwest	28	7	25	11	19	1	4	4	14	5	18
Southwest	66	5	8	21	32	2	3	12	18	26	39
Northwest	17	4	23.5	4	23.5	2	12	5	29	2	12
Total	382**	51		135		18		66		112	

*No schools were classified as medical model.

**Of the 417 schools, 35 returned unanswered questionnaires.

Table 3. Frequencies of each of three criteria for formulating nursing diagnoses obtained from 200 nursing care plans (categorized by curriculum category)

Curriculum category	Criterion #1 present	Criterion #2 present	Criterion #3 present
Systems n = 50	36	27	33
Developmental n = 50	28	18	28
Interaction n = 50	22	16	23
Mixed n = 50	25	7	14
Total N = 200	111 (56%)	68 (34%)	98 (49%)

Note: Total of all criteria met = 277 out of a potential 600.

in region 7, these fifteen represent 88% of the baccalaureate schools in that region. Region 2, with 50% of the schools responding, was the geographic area returning the smallest percentage of the total number of questionnaires sent to a region.

Categorizing baccalaureate schools of nursing by curriculum model was necessary for the successful completion of Phase II in which randomly selected schools from each curriculum category were asked to forward nursing care plans from senior students for the purpose of determining ability to formulate nursing diagnoses.

FINDINGS OF PHASE II

The three criteria previously mentioned were employed to determine formulation of a nursing diagnosis. A frequency distribution that summarizes the data with regard to the number of times one of each of three criteria was met in formulating nursing diagnoses is found in Table 3. In Table 4 a frequency distribution summarizes data with regard to the total number of criteria met by each subject and recorded on the nursing care plan.

Of the 200 nursing care plans analyzed, only 28% met *all* criteria for formulating nursing diagnoses and 35% met *none* of the three criteria. On the basis of these data senior students in baccalaureate schools of nursing are apparently seriously deficient in the ability to formulate nursing diagnoses. This deficit may be the lack of attention to detail in the problem-solving methodology as reported by Frederickson and Mayer.[19] Their study indicated that baccalaureate nursing students, although scoring high on critical thinking ability, did not use all steps of problem solving consistently and did not consider each step consciously.

Criterion #1 was most commonly met by nursing students. This criterion requires a description of nursing diagnoses in terms of client needs or client response rather

Table 4. Total number of criteria met for formulating nursing diagnosis obtained from nursing care plan (categorized by curriculum model)

Curriculum model*	None	Number of criteria met 1	2	All
Mixed	22	14	8	6
Interaction	21	8	11	10
Developmental	16	7	12	15
Systems	11	6	8	25
Total	70	35	39	56
N = 200	(35%)	(18%)	(20%)	(28%)

*No schools fell in the medical model.

than disease-centered or nurse activity to be performed. Of the nursing diagnoses formulated, 111 met criterion #1, which represented 56% of the nursing care plans analyzed. It appears from these data that senior nursing students are most familiar with and able to define an actual or potential health concern *of the client.*

Even though over half of the senior nursing students were able to define a client problem in terms of the client concern, specification of some measure of that concern was not demonstrated. Only 34% of the nursing diagnoses met criterion #2. Senior nursing students appeared to experience the most difficulty in specifying levels or extent of client concerns. Of particular note is the fact that students from mixed model schools demonstrated criterion #2 in only seven of the potential 50 nursing diagnoses. It will be recalled that mixed models are descriptive of schools whose curricula incorporate a combination of nursing theories and were found to score relatively high on medical model characteristics.

Criterion #3 was met by 49% of the 200 subjects in their formulation of nursing diagnosis. Of the nursing diagnoses that were client centered (meeting criterion #1), 88% stated concerns that could be altered or maintained through nursing interventions. The remaining 12% described client concerns that called for medical rather than nursing interventions. These data suggest that senior nursing students who define problems in terms of client concerns may be experiencing confusion with regard to the differences in practice between physicians and nurses. It is also possible that the data reflect the overlap that exists in the practice domain of physicians and nurses. Whatever the reasons, 12% of the students in this sample formulated medical rather than nursing diagnoses.

HYPOTHESIS 1: ANALYSIS OF THE DATA

It had been predicted that the systems model curricula would be more effective in preparing senior nursing students to formulate nursing diagnoses. An analysis of variance was performed on the data to test whether the four curriculum models

Table 5. Analysis of variance with number of criteria present as dependent variable

Source	df	SS	MS	F
Grand mean	1	383.65		
Model	3	27.9	9.3	2.59
School (M)	16	57.5	3.59	2.97*
Error	180	217	1.21	

*$p < .05$

resulted in differing levels of performance on the number of criteria met for formulating a nursing diagnosis. (Table 5.)

The effect of the curriculum model was not significant ($F = 2.59$, $p <$ 05). This failure to reject the null hypothesis implies that differences observed among curriculum models could well be due to chance. The findings also suggest that curriculum models in themselves are not differentiating variables when measured by diagnoses formulation ability.

The effect of nursing school nested within curricular model did prove to be significant ($F = 2.97, p < .05$). This implies that real differences exist among schools of nursing in the effectiveness with which they teach nursing diagnoses, differences that cannot be explained by the general curriculum model followed.

The initial hypothesis suggested that curriculum models would affect the ability of students to formulate nursing diagnoses and was based on the nursing literature, curriculum theory, and personal experience in education. Because of the fact that the findings of the study were in the hypothesized direction, the power of the analysis of variance F test was determined. The purpose of calculating the power is to determine the probability of making a Type II error in the decision process, which is failure to reject the null hypothesis when it is false. The power was calculated at $\phi = .30$, a 70% probability of a Type II error being committed. This low power suggests that the number of schools in the sample population was insufficient for the treatment effect to show significance. Thus it would be considered worthwhile to extend the study to a larger sample population of schools.

The frequency table (Table 4) shows the number of students incorporating each of the criteria in their care plans. The data are in the direction hypothesized, although that trend is not sufficient enough to be significant. Although this study has not demonstrated that the curriculum model is a variable that predicts ability to formulate nursing diagnoses, the fact still exists that some students are able to formulate nursing diagnoses and some are not.

These findings indicate that hypothesis 1, systems model curricula will significantly differentiate senior nursing students' ability to formulate nursing diagnoses, was not confirmed.

HYPOTHESES 2 AND 3: ANALYSIS OF THE DATA

It had been predicted that student-involved teaching strategies and essay-type

Table 6. Correlation coefficient between criteria met, teaching strategies, and assessment methods

Variable	Teaching strategies: Didatic	Teaching strategies: Student-involved	Assessment methods: Objective	Assessment methods: Essay
Criteria met	.17	.06	−.69*	.10
Didatic		.52*	−.44*	.17
Student-involved			−.04	.32
Objective				−.47*

$^*p < .05$

assessment methods would correlate positively with students' ability to formulate nursing diagnoses. A correlation matrix is shown in Table 6.

No significant correlation is found between student-involved teaching strategies and criteria met for formulating nursing diagnoses. Therefore null hypothesis 2 failed to be rejected. Further analysis of the data showed no significant correlation between didactic teaching strategies and criteria met, which seems to indicate that the ability to formulate nursing diagnoses is not affected by the strategies used by nursing professors. However, students report both didactic and student-involved teaching strategies are employed. Thus the moderately high correlation between both types of teaching strategies, lecture, group discussion, demonstration, and seminars are some of the strategies that students checked on the response form as frequently used in their nursing courses. These data seem to indicate a variety in teaching strategies although in this study that variation cannot be related to the ability to formulate nursing diagnoses.

No significant correlation is found between essay-type assessment and number of criteria met for formulating nursing diagnoses. Therefore null hypothesis 3 failed to be rejected. It should be noted that the correlation between criteria met and essay-type testing is in the expected direction. Further, a moderately high negative correlation was found between objective type assessment and number of criteria met. The value of r^2 for objective testing was .48 and was .01 for essay-type testing, which indicates that objective testing explains 48% of the variance. There was insufficient variation in essay-type testing to result in a significant correlation. Thus the expected direction in the correlation between essay testing and criteria met and insufficient variation because of few essay-type tests compared to objective type suggests that the relationship between the essay variable and criteria met for formulating a nursing diagnosis is still open to question.

The negative correlation between objective assessment and criteria met indicates that the fewer criteria met for formulating a nursing diagnosis, the more likely the

The fewer the criteria met for formulating a nursing diagnosis, the more likely the student will be assessed by objective tests.

student will be assessed by objective tests. It is possible that preparation for objective testing may not facilitate the skills required for formulating diagnoses. Matthews and Gaul[7,8] found that cognitive skills such as concept attainment and critical thinking are requisite for formulation of nursing diagnoses. The extent to which objective testing or preparation for objective testing assists students in developing these skills is a question worthy of further investigation.

The negative correlation with respect to objective testing and diagnoses formulation may indicate that deficiency in meeting criteria is undetectable in present objective testing. It is also possible that students who have deficits in formulating nursing diagnoses do poorly on objective testing. This study does not examine the extent to which this is true but raises the question for further study.

The significant negative relationship between objective and essay-type assessment indicates that frequent use of essay-type testing in schools of nursing preclude the frequent use of objective testing and vice versa.

The results of the analysis of the data from the student response form indicate that hypotheses 2 and 3 were not confirmed.

CONCLUSIONS

Ability to formulate a nursing diagnosis is not a demonstrated competence of senior nursing students, at least as found by this study. This finding may be indicative of the level of theory development surrounding nursing diagnoses or the extent to which diagnoses is used, understood, and taught by nursing faculty. Until each of these possibilities is investigated and curricula altered accordingly, students' abilities to formulate nursing diagnoses are likely not to improve.

Second, the models on which baccalaureate nursing curricula are developed differ. The extent to which these differences facilitate or retard the development of nurses' abilities to diagnose has not been demonstrated in this study. However, further study of curriculum models with senior student subjects may help to determine how differences in curricula with respect to content, process, and foci affect the effectiveness of the subjects' ability to formulate nursing diagnoses.

IMPLICATIONS FOR NURSING EDUCATION

Organizing and building a clinical science in nursing depends on identifying client health problems that are diagnosed and treated by nurses. The obvious assumption therefore is that competence in making an accurate nursing diagnosis is of major importance for the practice of nursing.

The results of this study seem to indicate a pervasive deficiency on the part of nursing students to make such diagnoses. This deficit may reflect the "state of the art" with regard to the development of diagnostic nomenclature. It may be explained in part by the ability of professors in nursing to teach diagnoses in that some professors may lack the requisite knowledge themselves. Or the observed deficit may be explained by the teaching framework used by professors of nursing as they assist students to derive nursing diagnoses from client data. Another possibility is that students find it difficult to apply theoretical knowledge to the practice setting. A further possibility may be that the profession's utilization of the concept of nursing diagnosis is not sufficiently developed to be transmitted consistently and clearly in teaching students. Whatever the reasons, this study raises a question that should be of concern to educators: Why are senior nursing students deficient in formulating nursing diagnoses?

Formulating a nursing diagnosis

The design of this study allowed gathering data on strengths as well as deficiencies in students' formulation of nursing diagnoses. Students in this sample are proficient in defining problems specific to the client. Nursing care plans analyzed for this study were generally client oriented and client focused.

However, students experienced difficulty in formulating a nursing diagnosis when attempting to define the levels of competence or dysfunction of clients. This specificity in the client problem or concern is a crucial aspect of diagnosis because it determines the type and amount of nursing intervention needed by the client. Without a specification of level, the evaluative step of the nursing process lacks a point of reference from which to determine the effectiveness of the intervention.

The findings of this study indicate that nursing students are deficient in meeting criterion 2 when formulating a nursing diagnosis, a finding that has implications for nursing education. Professors of nursing responsible for teaching and reinforcing use of the nursing process should consider teaching nursing diagnosis in a developmental fashion highlighting each step of the process. Further, assessment of nursing students should include types of testing that can determine whether needed skills for formulating nursing diagnosis have been learned as well as whether the theoretical understanding of each criterion has been achieved.

This study has implications for nursing far beyond the issue of diagnosis formulation. The nursing diagnosis is the problem-identification step of the nursing process. It is the pivotal point of nursing intervention. It is the major focus of client concern or need and it becomes, at the evaluation step, the criterion by which the effectiveness of nursing intervention is determined. Diagnostic ability therefore is necessary for effective professional nursing practice.

Clearly, effective practice includes nursing intervention that is not a "standard set of actions" but rather individualized activities determined by the professional nurse on the basis of the identified diagnosis. It follows then that the skill of formulating nursing diagnoses is a necessary requisite for intervention planning.

This study, which has demonstrated a deficiency in the ability of senior nursing students to formulate nursing diagnoses, raises a further educational question: Is the ability to formulate nursing diagnosis related to the ability to provide effective nursing intervention? A report of these studies can also be found in Matthews and Gaul.[20]

Teaching strategies and assessment instruments

A further result of this study indicates that teaching strategies are not significantly correlated with ability to formulate nursing diagnoses, although student respondents report that a variety of strategies are used in baccalaureate schools of nursing. This is true regardless of the type of curriculum. Although there are few studies in the literature correlating teaching strategies to measurable outcomes, Dubin and Taneggia[21] found "no measurable difference among methods of college instruction when evaluated by student performance on final examinations."(p35) This study of ability to formulate nursing diagnoses supports the 1968 findings of Dubin and Taneggia with respect to teaching strategies. Variations in teaching strategies do not seem to affect the quality of the students' performance when evaluated by ability to formulate diagnoses. Still the question must be raised: Are there certain teaching strategies that are more effective in teaching the skills necessary for the formulation of nursing diagnosis? If so, what are they? If not, why vary the teaching strategies?

Hypothesis 3 predicted that essay-type testing would be found more frequently associated with students who meet all criteria for formulating nursing diagnosis. The basis for this hypothesis were studies such as Matthews and Gaul,[7,8] who found cognitive skills of concept attainment and critical thinking necessary for nursing diagnosis; such skills may be demonstrated in essay-type assessment.

Students reported that both objective and essay-type testing are employed in baccalaureate schools of nursing. A moderately high negative correlation was found between objective testing and criteria met, which indicates that students who have difficulty formulating nursing diagnoses are most frequently assessed by objective testing. A major question for educators is raised by this finding: Is objective testing adequate for detecting deficiencies in ability to formulate nursing diagnoses?

A significant correlation was not found between essay-type testing and number of criteria met for formulating nursing diagnoses. These data suggest that students with high ability in diagnoses formulation are as likely to be assessed through essay-type testing as students with low ability.

These data indicate further that essay-type testing is an infrequent method of assessment used in baccalaureate schools of nursing. It is possible that this infrequent use resulted in the lack of significance seen in the data. The correlation of essay with criteria met was positive in the expected direction. The correlation of objective testing with criteria met was negative, also in the expected direction. Because of these findings, it is suggested that further investigation of this phenomenon be undertaken in a future study using an equal number of objective and essay-type assessments with an experimental and control group to determine the relationship between essay assessment and ability to formulate nursing diagnoses.

CURRICULUM MODELS

The data from this study indicate no significant relationship between types of curriculum models and students' ability to formulate nursing diagnoses. Thus the relative importance of curriculum model in baccalaureate nursing education is open to question.

There is a perception among nurse eduators that a majority of schools have substantially shifted to nursing models of curriculum. It appears from this study that the perceived change has actually taken place. This shift is most evident in problem-solving content where the focus has changed from disease problems to client problems.

The number of schools identified as systems model curricula (56%) suggests that nursing faculty are beginning to select this specific nursing model more frequently than others. The selection of a model or models to be used in education depends upon the goals of the curriculum and the preference of the nurse educators. The data from this study seem to indicate that systems models represent the ordered reality of nursing's focus (persons, the environment, and health) more clearly or perhaps more effectively for the nurse educators themselves. It is conceivable that these data indicate a shift toward a concrete, clinically useable conceptual model, developed from a combination or synthesis of the nursing models now in use.

REFERENCES

1. Goldmark J: *Nursing and Nursing Education in the United States.* New York, The Macmillan Co., 1923.
2. Yura H, Walsh M: *The Nursing Process.* New York, Appleton-Century-Crofts, 1978.
3. Feldman KA, Newcomb TM: *The Impact of College on Students: Summary Tables.* San Francisco, Jossey-Bass, 1969.
4. Gamson Z: Assuring survival by transforming a troubled program: Grand Valley State College, in Grant G, Elbow T, Ewens T, et al: *On Competence.* San Francisco, Jossey-Bass, 1979, pp 410–438.
5. Ewens T: Transforming a liberal arts curriculum: Alverno College, in Grant G, Elbow T, Ewens T, Et al: *On Competence.* San Francisco, Jossey-Bass, 1979, 259–298.
6. Pace CR: *Measuring Outcomes of College.* San Francisco, Jossey-Bass, 1979.
7. Gaul A: *Concept Attainment and Cue Perception in Nursing Diagnoses and Critical Thinking,* thesis. Texas Woman's University, Denton, Tex, 1978.
8. Matthews C: *The Relationship Between Nursing Diagnosis and Critical Thinking,* thesis. Texas Woman's University, Denton, Tex, 1978.
9. Bush HA: Models for nursing. *Adv Nurs Sci* 1:18–22, January 1979.
10. King IM: *Toward a Theory for Nursing: General Concepts of Human Behavior.* New York, John Wiley & Sons, 1971.
11. Orem DE: *Nursing: Concepts of Practice.* New York, McGraw-Hill, 1971.
12. Orlando IJ: *The Dynamic Nurse–Patient Relationship: Function Process Principles.* New York, GP Putnam & Sons, 1961.
13. Henderson V: *The Nature of Nursing.* New York, Macmillan, 1966.
14. Rogers ME: *An Introduction to the Theoretical Basis of Nursing.* Philadelphia, FA Davis, 1970.
15. Johnson DE: The behavioral systems model for nursing, in Riehl JP, Roy Sister C (eds): *Conceptual Models for Nursing Practice,* ed 2. New York, Appleton-Century-Crofts, 1980, pp 207–216.
16. Roy Sister C: *Introduction to Nursing: An Adaptation Model.* Englewood Cliffs, NJ, Prentice-Hall, 1976.
17. Neuman B: The Betty Neuman health care systems model: A total person approach to patient problems, in Riehl JP, Roy Sister C (eds): ed 1. New York: Appleton-Century-Crofts, 1974, pp 99–114.
18. Gebbie K, Larin M (eds): *Classification of Nursing Diagnosis.* St. Louis, The CV Mosby Co, 1975.
19. Frederickson K, Mayer G: Problem-solving skills: what effect does education have? *Am J Nurs* 77:1167–1169, July 1977.
20. Matthews AM, Gaul AL: Nursing diagnosis from the perspective of concept attainment and critical thinking. *Adv. Nurs Sci* 2:17–26, October 1979.
21. Dubin R, Taneggia JC: *The Teaching-Learning Paradox.* Eugene, Ore, Center for the Advanced Study of Educational Administration, University of Oregon, 1968.

Models and Model Building in Nursing

Wade Lancaster, M.B.A.
Assistant Professor of Marketing

Jeanette Lancaster, M.S.N., Ph.D.
Associate Professor
Community Mental Health Nursing
University of Alabama in Birmingham
Birmingham, Alabama

NURSING EDUCATION HAS historically focused on knowledge related to practice skills. However, in recent years increasing emphasis in the classroom has been placed on research and theory. Nursing has moved from an applied art borrowing theories from the behavioral and physical sciences to explain its practice to a profession actively involved in the delineation and development of nursing theory. Few topics are receiving more attention in the nursing literature than the need for a refined and clearly articulated theoretical base.

Nursing educators and practitioners generally agree that nursing theory, practice, and research are intimately interdependent. Theory can only be derived from research in nursing practice. Chinn and Jacobs maintain that "the development of theory is the most crucial task facing nursing today."[1(p1)] If nursing is to gain power and prestige within the health care system it is increasingly important that practitioners have theoretical bases for their practice.

As one way of moving toward the development of a theoretical base for practice Chinn and Jacobs[1] have set forth a four-stage set of operations for a theory development system: (1) concept examination and analysis, (2) formulation and validation of relational statements, (3) theory construction, and (4) the practical application of theory. While there is no argument with their position that nurses must become increasingly involved in the development of theory, the mastery of each step in this four-stage process needs careful attention. Chinn and Jacobs emphasize that concept examination and analysis is probably the most important, yet most frequently overlooked, operation in the theory development system.

A model is a device to facilitate the examination and analysis of concepts. Unfortunately not enough attention has been devoted (either in the classroom or in the literature) to the development of models. Students seem intimidated by the prospect of developing and using models in either practice or research. The purpose of this article is to define and classify models, outline the model building process, and discuss the advantages and disadvantages of models. The position taken here is that a basic understanding of both models and their development is a first step in the process toward theory development.

WHAT ARE MODELS?

Most people tend to view a model as any structure which purports to replicate, reproduce, or represent something else. While this notion of a model is consistent with the scientific view of a model, it ignores the use to which the model is put. Hence a key distinction between the common view of a model and the scientific view is in the use to which the model is put.

In the scientific sense a model may be used to define or describe something, to assist with analysis of a system, to specify relationships and processes, or to present a situation in symbolic terms that may be manipulated to derive predictions. There seems to be only one common characteristic of the various usages of scientific models. According to Kaplan, "we may say that any system A is a model of system B if the study of A is useful for the understanding of B without regard to any direct or indirect causal connection between A and B."[2(p263)]

In various branches of science, engineering, and industry models are used to solve both simple and complex problems by concentrating on some portion or some key features instead of on every detail of real life. This approximation or abstraction of reality, which may be constructed in various forms, represents the scientist's idea of a model. As Hazzard[3] points out, no one segment of the human universe is

Models are used to solve both simple and complex problems by concentrating on some portion or some key features instead of on every detail of real life.

so simple and easy to understand that it can be grasped and controlled without the use of abstraction. Consequently, models do not, and cannot, represent every aspect of reality because of the innumerable and changing characteristics of the real world to be represented. Because models use abstraction, attention is focused only on the details of reality that are perceived to have the greatest relevance to the situation. This feature is an intrinsic part of the scientific model.

RELATIONSHIP BETWEEN MODELS AND THEORIES

The term *model* has often been used as a synonym for theory. While many authors use these terms interchangeably, the substitution of one term for the other has led to their misuse. As Rudner notes, the term *model*, like the term *theory*, shows a "melancholic lack of uniformity in the vocabulary of scientists and others who talk about science."[4(p23)]

The position taken here is that all theories are models, because all theories purport to represent some aspect of real world phenomena. However, the converse is not true; all models are not theories because many models will not have all the requisites of theoretical construction. To qualify as a theory, the phenomena under consideration must be precise and limited, and the concepts need to be clearly defined.[5] Theory also includes the capability for prediction and control regarding the relational statements set forth about the phenomena which constitute the theory.[1] Hence, according to Rudner, "A theory is a systematically related set of statements, including some lawlike generalizations, that is empirically testable. The purpose of theory is to increase scientific understanding through a systematized structure capable of both explaining and predicting phenomena."[4(p10)]

While a model describes the structure of events or systems, a theory moves beyond description to the level of prediction by stating relationships among components. Models provide useful mechanisms for depicting the relationships which exist among the variables of the theory. The construction of a model allows theorists to graphically illustrate and explain relationships. In this context model building is viewed as an early step in the more time-consuming and complex process of theory development.

Although certain characteristics distinguish models and theory from one another, they also share certain common qualities. Both vary in their degree of abstractness, and both are isomorphic systems. Isomorphism refers to the similarity between a thing and model of it.[6(p580)] For a model to be maximally useful, it must accurately depict the object which it purports to represent. Isomorphism requires a one-to-one correspondence between the model or theory and reality. While models are an important tool for theory construction, not all models are designed for this purpose. Therefore to more fully understand the nature of models, they need to be classified.

CLASSIFICATION OF MODELS

Any model can be classified and described in different ways. However, the

Mental Image Models	Symbolic Models	Physical Models
(Highly abstract)		(Concrete, specific replicas)

Fig 1. Models classified according to level of abstraction.

task of categorizing models is complicated by the lack of a uniform terminology. A comprehensive review of the literature revealed a considerable variety of terms used to distinguish among various types of models. When several terms are used to describe the same type of model, confusion rather than clarification results. In the classification schema which follows, the basic types of models are identified and, where possible, synonymous terms are noted.

Classification according to level of abstraction

Models are frequently described according to their level of abstraction, which essentially refers to their composition or manner of presentation. When models are classified according to their level of abstraction, they can be arranged along a continuum with *mental models* at one polar end and *physical models* at the other. In this context mental models represent the highest degree of abstraction. In contrast, physical models are specific, concrete replicas of their real-life counterparts. Symbolic models are positioned between pure mental models and physical models. Thus by starting with mental models and moving toward physical models, all models can be positioned on a continuum in which the manner of presentation becomes less abstract (Figs 1 and 2).

Mental models

Mental models, sometimes called images or implicit models, are the pictures of the world held in the mind. Mental models consist of thought patterns composed of words and concepts arranged to constitute a meaningful image of reality. These thought patterns can be

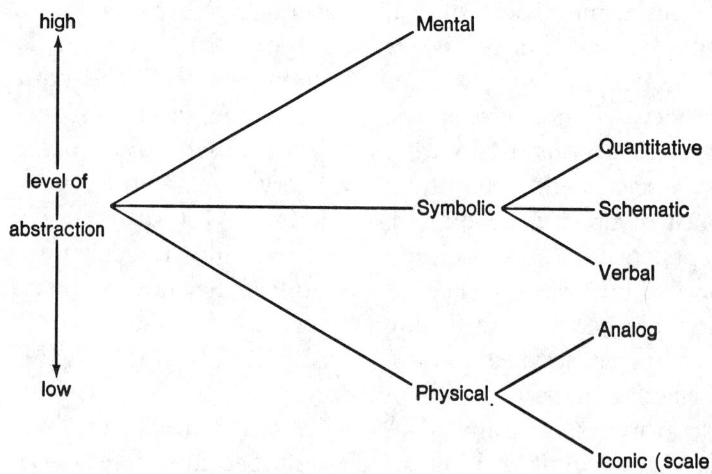

Fig 2. Classification of models according to level of abstraction and including subcategories.

formulated into language, which ultimately allows people to communicate and describe abstractions to others.

A mental model is a simplification of the situation it portrays, consisting of a few incomplete and abstract concepts which are considered integral to forming a meaningful image of reality. It is fortunate that mental models reduce the full scope of the situations which they portray. This enhances their usefulness by not overwhelming the individual with the complexities of reality. The real value of mental models comes from their not corresponding precisely to the complexity of the phenomenon under scrutiny. Instead the model focuses on the details of reality which have the perceived greatest relevance to the situation.

Physical models

Not all phenomena can be understood by the use of mental models. Consequently highly abstract models may become explicit in the form of physical models.

Iconic models. One type of physical model is the iconic model. An iconic model looks like what it is supposed to represent; it is a physical representation of some real-life object, either in a somewhat idealized form or on a different scale. Some iconic models are exact replicas of the entities they are designed to represent, whereas others deviate from reality in the number of properties represented. Iconic models are sometimes referred to as scale models. While not all iconic models involve a change in size, many are designed to be either smaller or larger than the entity being depicted.

Iconic models are frequently used by engineers and designers. For example, they are used in the design of ocean liners, bridges, water supply systems, and various products, ranging from automobiles to stage scenery. Aeronautical engineers use miniature models of airplanes to represent full-sized planes in wind tunnel tests. Iconic models are also used by nurses as replicas of various body organs, such as the heart, kidney, or brain, used for instructional purposes.

Analog model. When a model ceases to look like its real-life counterpart, thus becoming more abstract, while simultaneously retaining physical properties, it is referred to as an analog model. In contrast to iconic models, in analog models properties are transformed. One property is used to represent another. There is a substitution of components or processes to provide a parallel with what is being modeled.

A topographic map in which the property color is substituted for height above sea level is one common example of an analog model. Another example is a graph, such as an electrocardiogram (ECG), in which a unit distance along a line is used to represent a unit of time or speed. The ECG is realistic in behavior, reflecting what is occurring in the heart, but it does not have characteristic features of any aspect of the processes producing the data displayed.

Symbolic model

When a model no longer has a recognizable physical form and takes on a higher level of abstraction it becomes a symbolic model. In this type of model, phenomena are represented figuratively by using a set of connected symbols, objects, or concepts.[7] Symbolic models can be either verbal, schematic, or quantitative.

Verbal model. A *verbal* model is any worded statement indicating the important aspects of a phenomenon. It is either written or spoken in a language that is familiar to those who seek to understand the model.

An important characteristic of this type of symbolic model is that it is easily constructed and communicated. For example, in medicine effective verbal models that describe the transmission of disease have been useful in the eradication of many epidemic diseases. Similarly, Harvey's model of the circulatory system and the various models of the reaction of the human body to invading organisms have influenced the development of the modern treatment of diseases.

Schematic model. Another type of symbolic model is the schematic model, which represents a useful next step in the process of symbolizing a verbal model. Many diagrams, graphs, drawings, pictures, and similar schemata are schematic models. This type of model is more abstract than the analog model mentioned earlier. It is generally descriptive, but it cannot be easily tested for representativeness and may lack precision. However, schematic models often provide an effective way to communicate with nonexperts and can bring together ideas that will be used in formulating other types of models.

One common example of a schematic model is the communications map of an organization, such as a hospital, which uses arrows to show how messages and other means of communication are transmitted. The map does not show anyone talking to anyone else and yet one can easily determine from the map which persons communicate with each other.

Quantitative model. A final type of symbolic model is the quantitative model, which uses mathematical symbols to represent a phenomenon or certain aspects of a phenomenon. Such a model possesses many useful and desirable characteristics. Quantitative models are concise and add the potential for certain kinds of precision. Moreover, they are not easily misconstrued. Mathematical symbols are easier to see and manipulate than words because tools of logic and mathematics may be used with quantitative models. Finally, quantitative models are easier to test and replicate than other types of models.

There are various types of quantitative models, some of which are relatively simple while others are extremely complex. One example of a quantitative model is the health belief model, developed by Becker,[8] which has been expressed in the form of several equations as well as being depicted verbally and schematically.

CLASSIFICATION ACCORDING TO PURPOSE

Not only can models be distinguished from one another in terms of their level of abstraction, but one model can be contrasted with another by considering its purpose. The intent of the model brings into focus a variety of factors which have been used to distinguish various types of models. By using a series of bipolar adjectives, models can be categorized according to their purpose (Table 1). More specifically, models can be classified as being physi-

Table 1. Classification of models according to purpose

Category	Subcategory	Purpose
Physical		Represent structure
vs		
Behavioral		Depict performance
or		
Static		Portray phenomenon at a given point in time
vs		
Dynamic		Show time as an independent variable
or		
Micro		Focus on individual units and detailed linkages between variables
vs		
Macro		Use varying levels of aggregation and gross relationships between variables
or		
Partial		Limited to a few variables, developed in detail
vs		
Comprehensive		Identify many variables, developed in detail or linked with gross relationships
or		
Descriptive		Describe things as they are or as they act
	Communicative	Describe structural arrangement
	Explanatory	Describe causal relationships
	Predictive	Forecast future behavior or events
vs		
Decision		Find problem solutions
	Optimization	Find best solution
	Heuristic	Find a satisfactory solution

cal or behavioral, static or dynamic, macro or micro, comprehensive or partial, and descriptive or decision.

Physical versus behavioral models. When models are classified as being either physical or behavioral, the distinction is based on whether the purpose is to replicate the structure of a phenomenon or to duplicate its performance. For example, one purpose of using a model skeleton in an anatomy class is to show the structural relationship of the various bones in the skeletal system. In contrast, the purpose of two faculty simulating a nurse-patient encounter in the classroom is to demonstrate a behavioral phenomenon and illustrate to students a variety of intervention strategies.

Static versus dynamic models. A similar distinction can be made to differentiate between static and dynamic models. The purpose of a static model is to portray a phenomenon or group of phenomena at a given point. Static models do not readily portray change, although by using several or even a series of static models, change can be depicted. In contrast, dynamic models have time as an independent variable and emphasize the process by which change occurs.[9] For example, the life cycle concept is a dynamic model of human growth and development. In contrast, an organizational chart illustrates a static model. A set of photographs of a child at different ages represents a series of static models that could be viewed as a comparative dynamic model.

Micro versus macro models. Because models can be built at various levels of detail and complexity, another way of distinguishing among them is based on whether they are macro or micro. Models may be more or less aggregated in terms of the variables on which they build. The micro model is the least aggregated. Its purpose is to focus on individual units as well as to postulate detailed linkages between dependent and independent variables.[10(p618-619)] In contrast, the variables in macro or aggregated models may be of different kinds. Sometimes macro models use aggregated variables which are measured at the individual level, whereas other macro models use variables which have no counterparts at the individual level. While the micro model focuses on detailed linkages between variables, the purpose of macro models is to postulate two or more variables and link them with a gross set of relationships without explaining the specific mechanisms operating within each variable.[10(p618)]

An example of a macro model would be a description of the behavior of various population groups with regard to health care service utilization. In contrast, a micro model would focus on the health care service utilization behavior of an individual rather than an entire group.

Comprehensive versus partial models. Closely associated with macro and micro models are comprehensive and partial models. While these terms are occasionally used interchangeably, there appears to be a substantive difference between them. More specifically, comprehensive models attempt to identify and relate most or all of the variables involved in a phenomenon. These variables are then linked with a gross set of relationships, as is the case with macro models, or the variables are linked with more detailed relationships, as is the case with micro models.

Whereas comprehensive models attempt to identify most of the variables, partial models are limited to a few variables, but these variables are developed in detail. For example, a comprehensive model might examine individual health service utilization behavior by considering all possible variables such as demographic characteristics, and sociopsychological variables. In contrast, a partial model would be limited to the examination of selected variables such as attitudes toward health care services. Once again this examination might take place in either a micro or a macro context.

Descriptive versus decision models. Another way of classifying models, according to their purpose, is based on the distinction between descriptive and decision models. This distinction is frequently noted in the literature. However, terms such as *positive*, *systems*, *behavioral*, *empirical* and *concrete* have been used to refer to descriptive models. Similarly, terms such as *analytical*, *normative*, *goals*, *optimization*, *theoretical*, and *hypothetical* are often used to refer to decision models.

The general purpose of descriptive models is to describe things either as they are or as they work. Descriptive models can be broken down into three subgroups: communicative, explanatory, and predictive models. A communicative model describes the structural arrangement of the various elements or components in a system. An explanatory model describes the causal relationships among the elements in a system. The purpose of a predictive model is to assert or describe the causal relationships among the elements in a system before the events take place. Hence descriptive models either communicate, explain, or predict some phenomenon.[10(p618–619)] Freudian psychology and Maslow's hierarchy of human needs are examples of descriptive models.

In contrast to descriptive models, decision models propose how things should be. Decision models can be grouped into two categories: optimization models and heuristic models. Optimization models may have computational routines for finding the best solution to a stated problem. Examples of optimization models are differential calculus, mathematical programming, statistical decision theory, and game theory. Heuristic models are designed to evaluate alternative outcomes associated with different decisions and to find the best decision when optimization routines are not available or cost effective. Some heuristic models are referred to as rule-of-thumb approaches.[10(p620)]

In the preceding classification, models are categorized according to their purpose, in terms of a series of bipolar adjectives. By using one or more sets of bipolar adjectives (Table 1), any model can be described in terms of its purpose. If both classification schemes, level of abstraction and purpose, are combined, a relatively comprehensive means of classifying models is developed.

MODEL BUILDING

Model building allows for complex, real-world problems to be depicted visually, verbally, or quantitatively to assess relations among events, things, or properties. Some of these relational statements made possible by models are of a cause-and-effect nature.

Model building allows for complex, real-world problems to be depicted visually, verbally, or quantitatively to assess relationships among events, things, or properties.

Most real-world problems are complex and have an array of variables which affect their outcome. As a first step in systematically solving any problem, an individual should be able to describe, explain, or predict the pertinent part of reality through the use of abstractions such as thought processes, language, or pictures. Thoughts about any specific problem or situation are merely abstractions from reality. The abstractions which are made about a segment of reality are influenced by past experiences, perception, and the parameters of the current situation.

Thoughts or abstractions about a real situation may seem like three-dimensional moving pictures of the part of the real world that was perceived. The pictorial abstraction of reality frequently represents only a part of the total situation. Just as a photograph cannot capture the total range of hidden thoughts and beliefs, perceptions of reality are limited. Often the most critical and influential part of any mental image is that part which does not correspond to the concrete physical aspects of the situation. Model building and the process of abstraction allows part of reality to be represented at a given time by depicting complex events in a form which deletes extraneous factors and only portrays essential components of the situation.

Because model builders are concerned with phenomena which occur in the real world, the model builder must clearly describe the system which is to be analyzed. To describe the system that the model hopes to replicate, the model builder must clearly state the assumptions and values implicit in the model as well as in the society which comprises the environment for the model. For example, in a communications model, likely assumptions would include honest, straightforward interaction among participants, and the ability to hear as well as to understand the spoken or written word. Certain mechanisms for interchange would be implicit, including face-to-face contact, telephone, or the written mode of communication.

The model builder needs to maintain an awareness of the degree of congruence between the model and society at large or at least that segment of society which is in close influential proximity. For example, a model for open communications among all levels of an agency's hierarchy would be doomed to failure if the agency value was: "never talk to other departments or they will steal your ideas."

Next the model builder must be able to "observe and analyze a system of real events in order to isolate the determining variables that are operating in the system."[11(p8)] The major components of the model must be clearly defined and must also be identified as separate, observable units that can be related to one another.

To clearly and logically discuss the units of any given model the ultimate goal or outcome of the model must be described. Each variable or subset should be described in clear, easily understood terms which others can recognize and interpret. Next the actors in the model need to be noted as well as their expected roles and activities. For example, in a nursing situation the caregiver and recipient comprise the actors in the model; their roles, goals, and expected outcomes must be enumerated.

The next step is for the model builder to describe the goals and actual process of the steps taken or activities selected. The activities should relate to the problem statement, the expected outcome, and the characteristics of the actors. The choice of activities includes ongoing awareness both of the model's structure and its functioning because any alteration in one part of the model is likely to affect all other parts. The last skill for the model builder is clearly stating a set of defined concepts and statements which describe them as well as a set of statements which discuss the relationship between the concepts and constituent parts of the model.

Lippitt[12] elaborates on this last step when he purports that any model builder must describe thoroughly and accurately the situation, problem, or system by identifying the essential variables, components, or subsystems and then ask the following questions about each variable:

1. Relevance: Is each variable relevant and necessary for a clear assessment and understanding of the situation?
2. Relationships: How are the variables related to one another, to the total situation, and to characteristics external to the situation being scrutinized?
3. Relative importance: What is the weight of each variable according to

the magnitude of its significance to the total situation?

4. Outside constraints: What boundaries exist for the situation? What forces can exert an influence?
5. Internal constraints: What limits exist within the situation under consideration?

ADVANTAGES AND DISADVANTAGES OF MODELS

Positive and negative results can ensue from the use of models for depicting aspects of a practice-oriented profession such as nursing. The following advantages of models are set forth by Lippitt[12] and have transferability to nursing practice. First, models allow experimentation without risk. By using model building techniques a wide range of alternative interventions for any given problem can be addressed without actually altering the status quo. Such an approach takes a "what if" orientation. The model builder might initially set forth the current situation and then experiment with a variety of variables by considering: "What would be most likely to happen if I did ______?" The range of human reactions and responses to any change in the status quo cannot always be accurately predicted, but some ideas can be gleaned by considering the responses of the persons involved to previous change events.

A second advantage of using models, especially as a preliminary stage in the change process, is that models are good predictors of system behavior and performance. Models are more accurate as describers than as predictors. Any attempt at prediction must consider the wide range of human variables which could easily influence the outcome of the process.

A further advantage of model development for nursing practice is that models promote a higher level of understanding of the system than may have been previously held. To construct a model of a real world situation, careful attention must be paid to looking at each element as well as the relationships between them. By providing a careful assessment of the situation under consideration the model-building process promotes heightened awareness of the relative significance of each component. For example, if any change in A would most likely affect B, C, and then D, then A is central to the situation or problem being considered. Moreover, model building may often indicate where missing data exist. If a situation is being graphically depicted and there suddenly appears a gap in information, then the process has been useful.

The disadvantages inherent in model development may include a tendency to overgeneralize in an attempt to fit all the information available into a preestablished set of categories. The model builder may be tempted for the sake of simplicity and convenience to make the situation fit the model rather than trying to fit the model to the situation. Models have no truth in and of themselves; their accuracy lies in how well they describe reality. The lack of readily available evaluative tools also may be a disadvantage in model building. Once the model is built there may not be a clear-cut way to evaluate its effectiveness.

SUMMARY

There is considerable value in the nursing profession furthering its understanding of models. Nursing models are currently widely applied by both practitioners and academicians. The use of analogies, constructs, verbal descriptions of systems, idealizations, and graphic representations is widespread. As nurses become increasingly skillful at developing practice approaches based on sound theoretical information, the usefulness of models will increase.

REFERENCES

1. Chinn PL, Jacobs MK: A model for theory development in nursing. *Adv Nurs Sci* 1:1-11, October 1978.
2. Kaplan A: *The Conduct of Inquiry*. Scranton, Pa, Chandler Publishing Co, 1964.
3. Hazzard ME: An overview of systems theory. *Nurs Clin North Am* 6:385-393, September 1971.
4. Rudner R: *Philosophy of Social Science*. Englewood Cliffs, NJ, Prentice-Hall, 1966.
5. Williams CA: The nature and development of conceptual frameworks, in Downs FS, Fleming JW (eds): *Issues in Nursing Research*. New York, NY, Appleton-Century-Crofts, 1979, pp 89-106.
6. Brodbeck M: Models, meanings and theories, in Brodbeck M (ed): *Readings in the Philosophy of the Social Sciences*. London, Macmillan Co/Collier-Macmillan Limited, 1969, pp 579-600.
7. Hardy M: Theories: Components, development, evaluation. *Nurs Res* 23:100-107, March-April, 1974.
8. Becker MH (ed): *The Health Belief Model and Personal Health Behavior*. Thorofare, NJ, Charles B Slack, 1974.
9. Lazer W: The role of models in marketing. *Marketing* 26:9-14, April, 1962.
10. Kotler P: *Marketing Management*, ed 4. Englewood Cliffs, NJ, Prentice-Hall, 1980.
11. Stogdill R: Introduction—The student and model-building, in Stogdill R (ed): *The Process of Model-Building in the Behavioral Sciences*. Columbus, Oh, Ohio State University Press, 1970, pp 3-13.
12. Lippitt GL: *Visualizing Change: Model Building and the Change Process*. La Jolla, Calif, University Associates, 1973.

Ethics as a Component of Nursing Education

Marjorie Jones Stenberg, R.N., M.S., M.A.
Nurse-Epidemiologist
Veterans Administration Medical Center
Davis Park
Providence, Rhode Island

THOSE WHO WOULD add material or courses to the already burgeoning nursing curriculum should have compelling reasons for doing so. The nature of nursing practice, a rapidly expanding technology, a confusion of ethos and ethics within the profession, the multiplicity of nursing roles and the locus of decision-making power in others would seem to provide a basis for the inclusion of ethics in nursing education.

Although nurses function independently in many aspects of health care, they also practice their profession a great deal of the time in a unique "interface" situation between the patient and the physician. Amid the complex machinery at the bedside (calling for technical proficiency), the nurse (educated as a patient advocate) is serving as care-giver, administrator and coordinator but has little or no input into the major decisions made with or on behalf of the patient. "This combination of roles, very different from the physician's role, raises a host of ethical problems related to autonomy, coercion, role conflict, and personal identity."[1(p22)] And the failure of nurses to make meaningful contributions in patient care decision making may encourage the belief that ethical problems are also not part of their practice.

Nurses need part of their education devoted to making thoughtful, critical appraisals of what is ethical in daily practice and in policy development. They need to examine what Steinfels calls "the conflict between the professional model with which they are educated and the bureaucratic model under which they work."[2(p20)] Traditional medical ethics provides a poor fit with the unique problems nurses face in their practice. The inclusion of opportunities for ethics study as it relates to nursing is advantageous for both students and their future clients. Knowledge of adult moral development would seem to indicate that the years of professional education and early practice may be an ideal time for this study—especially if it is both comprehensive and relevant to practice.

THE STUDENT AND ETHICS

When planning ethics studies it is helpful to examine the stages of moral development and to build curricula based on the level of student attainment. Erikson and Piaget have examined moral thinking in children, but more interesting and to the point is the work of Kohlberg on stages in adult moral development.

When planning ethics studies it is helpful to examine the stages of moral development and to build curricula based on the level of student attainment.

Piaget questions the existence of adult stages and stage change in moral development. Stage change is defined as directed, sequential, qualitative transformations in psychological structure. Such change must be the result of experiential interactions with the environment rather than the result of normal biological maturation. Piaget postulates no new post adolescent cognitive stage, but Kohlberg thinks there are moral stages which first appear in young adulthood, as he has demonstrated in a longitudinal sample of individuals over 21.

Piaget's stage of formal operations may be said to coincide with Kohlberg's moral stage of social contract and utilitarian law making. To these, Kohlberg adds Stage 5B, or higher law and conscience orientation, and Stage 6, or universal ethical principle orientation. Kohlberg reports the attainment of principled moral reasoning in high school followed by "retrogression" to a skeptical egocentric relativism which is a transitional state between conventional and principled morality. He suggests that the nature of the experience leading to adulthood development, e.g., to principled moral thought, is somewhat different from that involved in childhood and adolescent movement through the conventional stages of moral reasoning. In childhood, there is an increasingly adequate comprehension of existing social norms and ideals developed through social and symbolic interaction. In contrast, construction of principles seems to require experiences of personal moral choice. "The crises and turning points in adult life are often of a moral nature, and literature describes dramas of maturity as the transformations of the moral ideologies of men."[3(p186)]

This view of adulthood moral stages linked to experience, besides being a rapprochement between Erikson's stage theory of development and a more cognitive structural stage theory, also indicates that moral development is taking place during much of the collegiate and professional educational years of nursing and medical students.

While most nursing education is social science oriented, considerable academic attrition in nursing programs comes from failure to meet the basic science requirements. Vaux has speculated that the student who is chosen for medical education (and increasingly for nursing) is one who excels in physics, chemistry, mathematics and biology—individuals who are quantitatively oriented and who "may be uniquely unsuited to think on affairs of the spirit and the heart."[4(pxiii)] Such individuals may develop science-oriented practice which ignores humanity and the problems of the patient. This idea and Kohlberg's work indicate a need for exploring ethics during health care education to provide a base for decision making that is broader than science alone.

PRESENTLY IMPLEMENTED PROGRAMS

The majority of the articles calling for ethics and humanities teaching for professionals have dealt with the subject in relation to medical schools. This attention to ethics arose slowly in the mid 1960s as a result of technological advances in patient care and the questions such care raised in the minds of both health care personnel and the public at large. Veatch and Sollitto, in a survey of such teaching presently established in American medical schools, report that of 107 schools responding, 97 indicated some kind of medical ethics teaching. Nineteen schools have only informal discussions, 56 offer special conferences, lectures or seminars and 47 have specific medical ethics electives. Only six have required courses, but faculty members with specific commitments to such teaching rose by 50% since 1972, from 19 to 31.[5]

The literature on teaching ethics to nurses is not extensive, and it is often concerned with professional adjustment, not ethics. Occasionally, articles appear in nursing journals about teaching ethics to medical students. An article purporting to discuss "the responsibility of the professional school for preparing nurses for ethical, moral and humanistic practice"[6] is really concerned with modification of practice, reform of systems of care and the "gate-keeper role" of the school in determining who gets into health careers.

In a recent review of the extent of ethics teaching in nursing schools, Aroskar reports data from 86 programs, 23% of which are on the baccalaureate level. Only six schools require a course in medical ethics, but 80% of the respondents have some planned curricular content on ethics. The average amount of time given this material is six to ten hours a year; most of the experience is in the junior and senior years. More frequently, respondents emphasized that, in some form, ethics is a component of every course in nursing. In addition, 50% of these programs offer out-of-class opportunities for ethics study in the form of workshops, symposia or faculty-student discussion groups. Fifteen schools responding have no planned opportunities for ethics studies; four of these do not feel a need for this subject in the nursing curricula.[7]

There are two authors who deal extensively with the methodology for teaching ethics: Bergman, who gives an example of an ethics course taught at the post-basic level at the University of Tel Aviv, and Baker, a social scientist who teaches at N. E. London Polytechnic.

Bergman believes that "ethical decisions are primarily a cognitive process and should be taught in nursing education programmes at all levels."[8(p140)] She has developed a model of the process involved in dealing with complex ethical issues. (See Figure 1.)

This is a logical pattern which follows the nursing process closely. The presenting situation is identified, the facts are gathered and the clarified situation is filtered through the individual's philosophy and knowledge, at which point the individual considers the options and makes a decision. The action taken is then evaluated and becomes part of a set of generalizations which can be used in a set of similar situations in the future.

In presenting this course, Bergman uses formal theoretical lectures, group discussion of content and methods, a review of nursing codes, and situational problems. As a basis for group discussion the following guidelines are used.

1. What facts are known?
2. What are the ethical problems (conflicts)?
3. What decisions are necessary before action can be taken?
4. Are there alternative courses of action?
5. What statements in the International Code for Nurses are relevant?

Baker presents a course which is also given in a post basic program. The subject

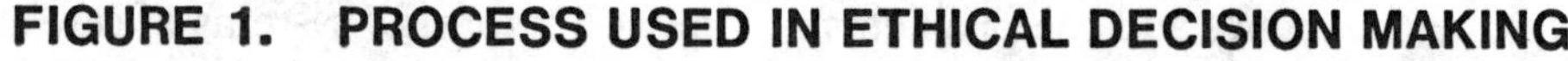

FIGURE 1. PROCESS USED IN ETHICAL DECISION MAKING

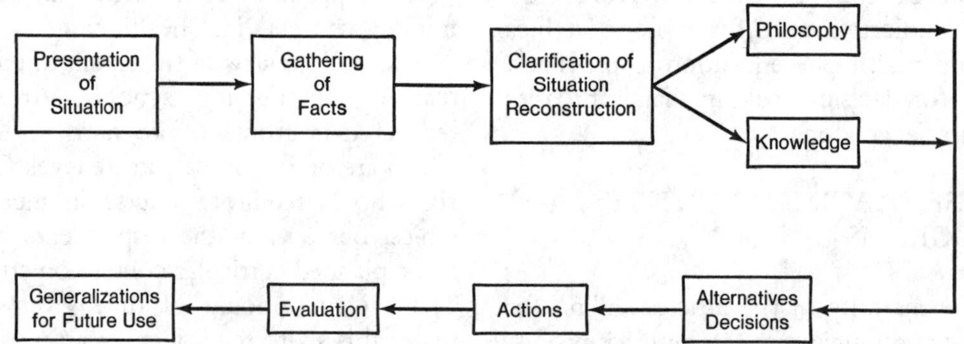

Source: Bergman, R. "Ethics Concepts and Practice." *Internat Nurs Rev* 20:5 passim (November-December 1973) p. 140.

is not included in the students' examinations, thus relieving one source of stress on the students. His principal objective is "to teach nurses how to think about something in which, so to speak, they are experienced practitioners since ethical decisions are in reality a daily activity."[9(p683)] He feels it is important for nurses to study ethics at its fullest sense of moral philosophy and not in the narrower sense of professional behavior.

To do this, Baker relies on the socratic exchange rather than on formal lectures. The exploratory stage, where students are questioning the meaning of words like "good" and "right," is the most difficult; it is often particularly hard to make the transition to the stage of analysis. Baker attempts to help students discover that behind every moral theory lies a theory of human nature. He also tries to help nurses look carefully at the unquestioning obedience they have been expected to give to authority. Baker contends that nurses bring so much to the study of ethics—problems not simply of exposition, but of substance for which the available text books are inadequate and remote from experience. "Teaching ethics to nurses is a remarkable way of compelling the philosopher to realize the shortcomings of his own subject."[9(p684)]

THE FRAMEWORK FOR TEACHING ETHICS IN NURSING EDUCATION

There is no question that ethics courses are not going to make individuals or institutions ethical; but the fact remains that exposure to ethics during professional

Exposure to ethics during professional education can establish a habit of thought or a technique of approaching patient problems which takes greater consideration of individual rights and needs.

education can establish a habit of thought or a technique of approaching patient problems which takes greater consideration of individual rights and needs. Bahm considers ethics a behavioral science which can be taught effectively by some of the techniques used in other behavioral sciences.[10] Ideally, ethics teaching should be begun in the early grades and, at the very least, by high school. Some medical schools may wish to require a formal ethics course before admission.

If ethics is to be taught in nursing education, differing frameworks must be considered: integration within the curriculum at all levels, a separate course as a requirement or an elective, or a combination of these two options. In order to integrate ethics throughout a nursing curriculum both a strong, unified commitment from the faculty and preparation of the faculty in techniques of integration of this particular subject are required.

If Kohlberg is correct, the nursing student's ethical development is an ongoing process. The integrated curriculum takes advantage of this to build even more complex and expanding viewpoints as the exposure to clinical situations increases. While integration of all content is a popular modality in nursing education, this approach may mean the neglect of some teaching, the haphazard placement of material in inappropriate sequence, or the failure to evaluate the teaching. "If ethics is to be considered a rigorous discipline in which students should study schools of thought, learn certain facts, and read and reflect on various problems, then a more specific course with well-prepared teachers and curriculum structure is necessary."[11(p25)]

The separate course framework immediately raises the question of who should teach ethics in a nursing curriculum. Should students be required to get their philosophical basics in a course in the philosophy department and then study ethics in the nursing curriculum? The courses now required by nursing from other departments are extensive; if ethics is taught exclusively outside of nursing, it may become of only peripheral interest to students. Competent humanists may be poor teachers in the nursing setting if they lack experience of the environment in which nurses practice.

Banks and Vastyan propose a new blending of humanistic and medical expertise in those who teach medical ethics. They also recommend that such teaching remain in the professional school to give it added validity with students.[12] It would probably be advantageous to place such a course in the senior year to take advantage of the maturity of students, their greater clinical experience and their proximity to embarking on their careers. Veatch and Sollitto have made the interesting observation that "a crucial conceptual shift takes place when a medical school stops treating ethics as something that ought to permeate the curriculum and begins to systematically plan its offerings. An even more significant conceptual break occurs when the school stops thinking of the teaching as a course and begins to see medical ethics or related subjects as a program to be developed with institutional structure."[5(p1031)] Perhaps the path of development for the teaching of ethics in nursing will be from integration to course to program as it has been in many of the medical schools.

THE OBJECTIVES OF TEACHING ETHICS

The objectives for the teaching of ethics and much of the content will be the same no matter which type of teaching is chosen. Students should be encouraged to write their own objectives in addition to those of the instructor or the team. Suggested objectives might include:

The student will:

1. understand his/her own values and their sources;
2. be familiar with classical philosophical theory of ethics;
3. demonstrate the ability to identify ethical problems (conflicts) in several situations;
4. develop a personal philosophy of ethics as a framework for nursing interactions.

A MODEL FOR CONTENT

A model for content has been developed using curriculum material which would be satisfactory for both integration and a course. It is directed at assisting the students to incorporate ethics into their

FIGURE 2. MODEL FOR ETHICS TEACHING WITH EXTERNAL INPUT AND POSSIBLE OUTCOMES

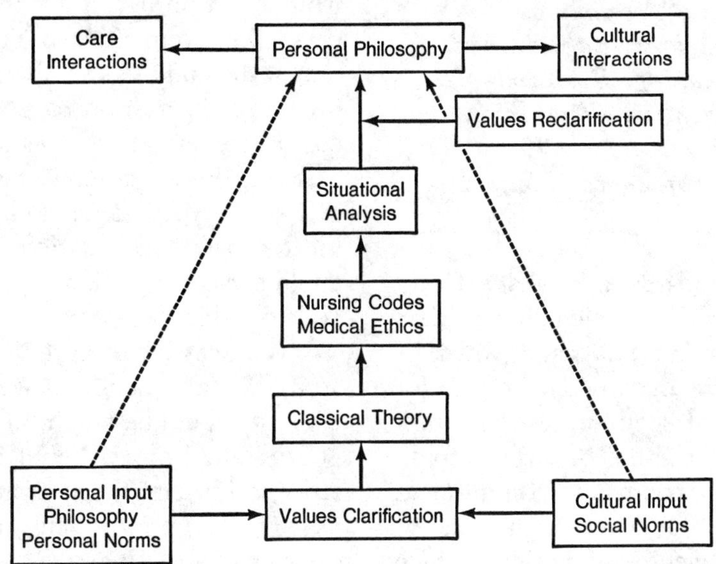

professional lives. (See Figure 2.) This model includes external input over which the instructor has little control, and expected outcomes (dotted lines). The model demonstrates the belief that personal and cultural input will still have a considerable direct effect after a formal study of ethics.

A basis for beginning ethics teaching should include values clarification seminars as developed by Simon, Howe and Kirschenbaum.[13] There is a need for an "educational experience whereby the student may gain clarity regarding values he holds, internal consistency between values and actions, and an adequate conceptual framework for decision making."[14(p251)] Values clarification can be done again at the end of the experience to illuminate change and growth for the student.

An introduction to classical ethics philosophers would follow values clarification, with readings selected from Plato, Cicero and others. A look at conscience through the work of Butler and Freud, the common-good theories of Mill and Bentham, Kant's theories of the formulation of moral obligation and respect for persons, a knowledge of Spinoza and the determinists who deny the possibility of freedom of human action, the philosophies of Hobbes and the Egoists, and Hume's concepts of humanity should be used as a basis for looking at the growing literature expressly concerned with medical ethics.

The study of nursing codes should be included specifically to demonstrate their limitations in ethical decision making. Even though they are frequently called ethics, nursing codes are primarily concerned with professional behavior. Such

The study of nursing codes should be included in ethics curricula to demonstrate their limitations in ethical decision making. Even though they are frequently called ethics, nursing codes are primarily concerned with professional babavior.

professional standards are what Haring terms "ethos" or that "which characterizes a professional culture ... and which is worked out in the occupational group for the fulfillment of their professional task and vocation."[15(p16)] Ethos begins in a tradition of sharing customs, a "commitment to particular values ... dedicated to increasing knowledge and skill, which originates with the profession."[15(p24)] Ethics, on the other hand, goes beyond ethos by addressing itself "to professional standards of human relationships, to a morality which permits living to the fullness of (one's) ethos."[15(p25)]

Only three of the eleven points of the American Nurses' Association's code for nurses can be considered ethics: (1) service with respect for human dignity, (2) patients' rights to privacy and protection, and (3) the safeguarding of the patient from the incompetent, unethical or illegal actions of others. The other eight statements are ethos; thus nurses have little to guide them in thinking through ethical problems. The International Code for Nurses, adopted in May 1973, has even less of a truly ethical orientation. There is an introductory statement that inherent in nursing is "respect for the life, dignity, and the rights of man unrestricted by considerations of nationality, race, creed, colour, age, sex, politics or social status."[16(p24)] This is a good philosophy of ethics, but aside from a section having to do with holding personal information in confidence, the rest of the code sets standards of behavior for nurses in relation to practice, society, coworkers and the profession in general. The guidelines written for nurses in clinical and other types of research have a much greater ethical orientation, and probably could serve as a basis for producing a real code of ethics.

It is interesting to note that in Aroskar's study, when respondents were asked what content should be taught in nursing ethics courses and how it should rank in importance, half (41) thought professional codes were a first priority; five others ranked them second. This may, as the author thought, indicate that professionals place great emphasis on the inculcation of professionalism in students. It is also possible that those faculty replying to the question have a misconception concerning the nature of the code and its relationship to ethics.

Situational analysis can best be accomplished with case studies which may be teacher prepared, those developed in the medical and nursing literature, or in student experience. Case studies provide excellent opportunities to examine patient/family rights, human experimentation, informed consent, truth telling and other major issues in health care. This type of study can be enhanced by using guideline questions such as those suggested by Bergman.

At the same time, students should be introduced to the highly critical reading of medical, nursing and biological research papers. As conscious as we think we are of human rights, papers appear with dismaying frequency about which serious reservations are in order. Gathering material for study and analysis has been a problem for many instructors. They may wish to examine Veatch's article in the June 1978 *Hastings Center Report* which is a review of recently published anthologies on bioethics.[17] A very valuable beginning text is *Moral Dilemmas in Medicine: A Coursebook in Ethics for Doctors and Nurses.*[18]

TEACHING ETHICS—AN EDUCATIONAL CHALLENGE

There is still the question of whether ethics can be "taught" at all. Perhaps it cannot be taught in the usual sense of that term. However, that the effort should be made is now widely accepted by educators in the health care professions. Attempts to evaluate ethics instruction will be very difficult; real evaluation may have to wait until this generation of medical and nursing students are practicing and doing research. Teaching ethics to nursing students presents an educational challenge in two dimensions: preparing cross-disciplined educators and developing a comprehensive, challenging, compassionate curriculum which meets the needs of the students and the patients for whom they will care.

REFERENCES

1. Jameton, A. "The Nurse: When Roles and Rules Conflict." *Hastings Center Rep* 7:4 (August 1977) p. 22–23.
2. Steinfels, M. O. "Ethics, Education, and Nursing Practice." *Hastings Center Rep* 7:4 (August 1977) p. 20–21.
3. Kohlberg, L. "Continuities in Childhood and Adult Moral Development Revisited" in Baltes, P. B. and Schail, K. W., eds. *Life-Span Developmental Psychology: Personality and Socialization* (New York: Academic Press 1973) p. 186.
4. Vaux, K. *Biomedical Ethics* (New York: Harper & Row 1974) p.xiii.
5. Veatch, R. M. and Sollitto, S. "Medical Ethics Teaching: Report of a National Medical School Survey." *JAMA* 235:10 (March 8, 1976) p. 1030–1033.
6. Shetland, M. L. "The Responsibility of the Professional Schools for Preparing Nurses for Ethical, Moral and Humanistic Practice." *Nurs Forum* 8:1 (1969) p. 17–28.
7. Aroskar, M. "Ethics in the Nursing Curriculum." *Nurs Outlook* 25:4 (April 1977) p. 260–264.
8. Bergman, R. "Ethics Concepts and Practice." *Internat Nurs Rev* 20:5 (November-December 1973) passim p. 140–141, 152.
9. Baker, E. "On Teaching Ethics to Nurses." *Nurs Times* 69:21 (May 24, 1973) p. 683–684.
10. Bahm, A. J. *Ethics as a Behaviorial Science* (Springfield, Ill.: Charles C. Thomas, Publisher 1974).
11. Aroskar, M. and Veatch, R. M. "Ethics Teaching in Nursing Schools." *Hastings Center Rep* 7:4 (August 1977) p. 23–26.
12. Banks, S. A. and Vastyan, E. A. "Humanistic Studies in Medical Education." *J Med Educ* 48:3 (March 1973) p. 248–257.
13. Simon, S., Howe, L. W. and Kirschenbaum, H. *Values Clarification: A Handbook of Practical Strategies for Teachers* (New York: Hart Publishing Co. 1972).
14. Dubos, R. *Man Adapting* (New Haven, Conn.: Yale University Press 1965) p. 251.
15. Haring, B. *Medical Ethics* (Notre Dame, Ind.: Fides Publishers 1973).
16. International Council of Nurses. "Code of Nurses: Ethical Concepts Applied to Nursing." *Internat Nurs Rev* 20:5 (November-December 1973).
17. Veatch, R. M. "Medical Ethics Anthologies: Alternatives for Teaching." *Hastings Center Rep* 8:3 (June 1978) p. 14–16.
18. Campbell, A. V. *Moral Delimmas in Medicine: A Coursebook in Ethics for Doctors and Nurses* (Edinburgh, London and New York: Churchill Livingstone 1975).

ADMINISTRATION, POLITICS AND EDUCATION

The Nursing Education Administrator: Accountable, Vulnerable, and Oppressed

Gertrude Torres, R.N., Ed.D.
Assistant Chairperson and Professor
Division of Nursing
D'Youville College
Buffalo, New York
Former Dean
School of Nursing
Wright State University
Dayton, Ohio

What can they do
to you? Whatever they want.
They can set you up, they can
bust you, they can break
your fingers, they can
burn your brain with electricity,
blur you with drugs till you
can't walk, can't remember, they can
take your child, wall up
your lover. They can do anything
you can't stop them
from doing. How can you stop
them? Alone, you can fight,
you can refuse, you can
take what revenge you can
but they roll over you.

But two people fighting
back to back can cut through
a mob, a snake-dancing file

This article is based on a presentation made at the National League for Nursing-American Association of Colleges of Nursing conference, Jackson Hole, Wyoming, July 21, 1980.
Poem reprinted with permission from Piercy M: The Moon Is Always Female. *New York, Alfred A Knopf, 1980.*

can break a cordon, an army
can meet an army.

Two people can keep each other
sane, can give support, conviction,
love, massage, hope, sex.
Three people are a delegation,
a committee, a wedge. With four
you can play bridge and start
an organization. With six
you can rent a whole house,
eat pie for dinner with no
seconds, and hold a fund raising party.
A dozen make a demonstration.
A hundred fill a hall.
A thousand have solidarity and your own newsletter;
ten thousand, power and your own paper;
a hundred thousand, your own media;
ten million, your own country.

It goes on one at a time,
it starts when you care
to act, it starts when you do
it again after they said no,
it starts when you say We
and know who you mean, and each
day you mean one more.

The Low Road
Marge Piercy

DEANS OF NURSING have the right and the obligation to facilitate professional nursing standards through the control of the educational program. Deans of nursing are primarily accountable *to* students (who represent the future of nursing as a profession), and *to* the health care consumer. It is this obligation of accountability that leads to vulnerability. It is in the best interest of nursing to clearly envision the dean's choices of accountability and to make these choices in a way that will overcome the more pervasive forces of oppression that inhibit realization of human potential in nursing. For the purposes of this article, *university* is used synonymously with *college* or other terms indicating the institution in which the nursing academic unit is housed; *deans* with *chairperson* or other terms indicating the administrator of the nursing academic unit; and the female gender is used in recognition of the fact that almost all deans of nursing are women.

THE HISTORY OF ACCOUNTABILITY AND CONTROL IN NURSING

At the heart of the problem of accountability and vulnerability is the fact that nurses often forget to whom the profession is accountable. The inability today of the profession to control nursing education and practice, to truly exercise accountability to students and health care clients, has deep historical roots in nursing. The need for women to develop their own potential and the related concern for nursing to control its own destiny were primary concerns of Florence Nightingale during her years of founding professional nursing. Nightingale clearly articulated the need for women to develop their passion, intellect, and moral activity and the need for nursing to maintain autonomy and control over its own destiny as a discipline distinct from that of medicine.[1-3]

Following Nightingale's philosophy, several nursing schools were established in the United States as autonomous educational programs. Kock described how

Annie Goodrich lost the autonomy of the nursing education program at Bellevue, which was founded on Nightingale's model:

> In 1895, as a result of the financial problems and the problems of administering a separate school, the board of directors of the hospital decided to take over the control of the training school and establish it as an integral part of the institution. This step constituted one of the most important deviations in the Nightingale system in America and one which has been the cause of many of the problems which have arisen for nursing educators ever since.[4(p28)]

Shryock, writing about the history of nursing, concluded that both the Bellevue School and the New Haven School lost their autonomy because of financial difficulties.[5] However, a more recent historical analysis of these and other schools founded on the Nightingale model reveals that the overt problem of financial difficulty was rooted in the basic problem of autonomy for the school of nursing and the desire of more powerful and financially stronger groups to control nursing education.[6]

The intimate connection between alleged "financial difficulties" and "autonomy" for nursing education is recorded in remarkable detail in the historical records of the Cincinnati Training School of Nurses, founded in 1888. In a recent historical study of this school Bruhn[6] found that the school closed in 1896 because it could not renew the contract with the Cincinnati General Hospital for student learning experiences. The Board of Trustees of the hospital was faced with a financial crisis in the hospital and viewed the financially solvent school as a means to achieving financial solvency for the hospital. The Board insisted that if the leaders of the school would not agree to a merger under the authority of the hospital board, the students would be barred from clinical learning experiences. The nursing leaders would not agree to the school's superintendent becoming an employee of the Board, the school closed, and the hospital later opened its own school of nursing. This trend continues despite growing evidence supporting the need for autonomous nursing programs.

The current literature abounds with stated beliefs and mandates directing members of the nursing profession to dictate the future of the profession rather than being controlled by other individuals and groups. The current movement began with Brown who recommended in 1951 that deans and faculties of nursing insist on full academic autonomy as a distinct discipline within the university setting.[7] Bridgewater, supporting this position, stated in 1979 that "a nursing unit which lacks autonomy is stifled in its contribution of meaningful input to the total university. Such a unit also fails to attract well-qualified, innovative faculty who are challenged to find employment in autonomous, professionally progressive programs."[8(p6)] Aydelotte, in a recent issue of *American Nurse,* predicted that the critical issue of the 1980s will be related to nurses' exerting control over their practice and their professional affairs.[9(p4)] As Ozimek states in projecting the future for nursing in the year 2000: "To remain a viable entity nursing must become independent, maintaining its autonomy and control of its own destiny."[10(p17)]

THEORETICAL FRAMEWORK OF OPPRESSION

The history of nursing and the situation of nursing as a profession today are consistent with the theoretical position of Freire,[11] whose basic premise is that a central problem for humanity is the historical evolution of a state of oppression or the objective exploitation of one person or group of people by another. The following basic propositions of Freire's theory are particularly applicable to the profession of nursing:

1. Realization of full human potential is a basic vocation for human individuals and groups.

2. Negation of humanization occurs by acts of injustice, exploitation, and dominance and leads to a yearning for freedom and justice. Such negation is a tacit acknowledgement of the human potential of the dominated group.

3. The oppressed state creates a distortion of reality for both the oppressed group and the oppressor group, in that the consciousness of the more powerful and privileged oppressor group is absorbed and taken to represent reality in the world. That is, the powerful group tends to identify the values and structure of society, the worthwhile goals, and the means of reaching these goals. This distortion leads to dehumanization for both the oppressed and the oppressor groups.

4. Only the group that is negated or oppressed can liberate itself and its oppressors, a process that begins with perceiving the state of oppression and becoming committed to action and thoughtful reflection (praxis) aimed toward becoming more fully human. Liberation will not be initiated or supported by the dominant group.

5. The barriers to liberation or to achieving freedom and justice are primarily rooted in the consciousness of the oppressed. These barriers include the oppressed group's internalized image of the oppressor as "powerful," "right," or "good"; the internalization of the consciousness of the oppressor (the oppressor's view and definition of reality); the oppressed group's fear of freedom; the tendency to conform to the prescribed behaviors set forth by the oppressor and to become in turn the oppressor; and the inability to take risks in achieving freedom.

6. Because it is in the perceived best interest of the powerful group to maintain its privileges, and its privileges depend on the continued domination of the less powerful group, the oppressed use various devices to assure continued domination. These devices include limiting the quality and extent of education granted the oppressed group, keeping the oppressed group divided among themselves, and granting periodic acts of false generosity for the oppressed groups. Acts of false generosity take the form of token rewards for continued loyalty to the goals of the dominant group, elevating a member of the oppressed group to a high-status position or giving verbal commendations and recognition for the labor of the oppressed group. These actions increase and become intensified whenever the dominated group begins to exert effort in the direction of freedom.

7. Actions to achieve liberation usually begin with acts that appear to be violent to the oppressor group but are essential to

Deans of nursing, as accountable leaders in the profession, are in particularly sensitive positions when viewed from a framework of oppression.

initiate control by the oppressed group of their own destiny and to claim their right to be liberated. The fight to be free is actually an act of love for the humanity of all people and focuses on changing the unjust social order to a system of accountability to all people.

Deans of nursing, as accountable leaders in the profession, are in particularly sensitive positions when viewed from a framework of oppression. They are identified by the dominant groups as their direct link to the educators and students of the profession and may in fact be placed in the position as an act of generosity by the dominant group. At the same time, deans are viewed as members of the profession by nursing educators and students. As their leaders they expect the deans to represent their best interests to the dominant group. The accountability of deans to each of these groups and to society at large and their vulnerability to oppressive forces are the focus of this article.

CONTROL OF NURSING EDUCATION AND PRACTICE

Control is an important concept to examine in relation to accountability and vulnerability because it is essential to one's own destiny or the destiny of the profession. The concept of control conveys a sense of restraining oneself, yet it is also related to having power and influence over others. The exercise of control over one's own self or one's own destiny can involve the contradictory dimensions of discipline, freedom, and power. This control must exist if one is to be accountable to someone, as well as the ability to justify and explain the needs of educational programs based on the demands of the discipline. It requires the power to manage nursing education and practice without unreasonable restraint. This control does not seek to extend the boundaries of control to other disciplines, although the need to influence related disciplines is essential.

Today administrators of academic units in nursing are not usually conscious of the inherent relationship between control of nursing education and control of nursing practice. Deans and faculties of nursing are deluded into thinking that the educational program is autonomous and free from the dominance of outside groups if the program gains token and illusionary autonomy within the structure of the academic institution. Regardless of academic structure, the dominance of nursing practice (particularly by medicine and hospital administrators) creates a source of control of the educational program. Thus deans and faculty lose their full ability to be accountable to students and to health care consumers.

Faculties of nursing work in classroom and clinical learning facilities that reflect a compromise with the standards of the profession. They are unable to educate within the true meaning of academic freedom and are compromised in their ability to maintain the professional integrity of nursing. Whenever faculties and deans choose to become more accountable and in control of nursing education and nursing practice, they are subject to increasing attack by outside groups who are attempting to maintain control of the profession. The conflict arising from such confrontations is an essential ingredient in changing the basic structure of the professional social order and will lead to healthier outcomes as long as members of the nursing profession remain committed to reclaiming control of their destiny.

DEFINITIONS AND PERCEPTION OF QUALITY

One measure of reality that is frequently used to justify and defend control of nursing education and nursing practice is the definition of quality. All concerned groups, including students, health care clients, nursing educators, nursing service personnel, physicians, hospital administrators, and university administrators are concerned with quality of the nursing education program. Because these viewpoints may not be congruent, providing a quality program becomes a major challenge.

Academic viewpoint

From the university's viewpoint, a dean's ability to provide a quality education is based on the ability to recruit and retain faculty who hold credentials consistent with the standards of the university. Such faculty must demonstrate a commitment to research and publication as well as excellence in teaching. This expectation leaves nursing programs open to attack. With the present limited availability of qualified educators in nursing, universities can readily claim that nursing as a profession is not ready to meet the challenges and demands of the academic environment as autonomous educational units.

This state of affairs continues to leave nursing deans in a particularly vulnerable position for token generosity granted by institutions of higher learning. These tokens take the form of either lowering the standards of academic qualifications for nursing programs commensurate with the general level of academic qualifications available among prospective nursing faculty or supporting the appointment of better qualified scientists from other disciplines to assist the nursing program. In either case the strength of the nursing unit is compromised.

Whittemore, discussing faculty survival, wrote that no profession can be saved unless its faculty are empowered to accept responsibility for their own destiny, including the maintenance of professional integrity.[12] Given this dilemma, deans of nursing who maintain a commitment to professional integrity for nursing will exert the primary effort in developing a sense of power among their faculty groups—recruiting well-qualified faculty and guiding all faculty in developing their academic potential.

Community expectations

The expectations of the community for quality in nursing programs often differ considerably from those of the academic environment. The community includes both the health care consumer and the consumer who employs the graduate of the nursing program. These consumer groups want graduate nurses who fit the image of the nurse that they believe will function effectively within the health care system. These groups expect production of practitioners at the lowest possible cost in the shortest possible time.

That portion of the nursing community that accepts the public image of the nurse wants a nursing graduate who is a "finished product," capable of functioning fully in today's hospitals and exhibiting behaviors based on the same set of values held by the general public. This image is reinforced by the demands coming from outside groups controlling nursing practice and is sometimes espoused by members of the nursing profession who represent interests other than that of the profession.[13] All of the demands coming from these groups may not necessarily be inconsistent with the standards of the profession, but the utilitarian goals and purposes of such demands require critical reflection by nursing educators and deans.

The nursing education profession and the standards set by leaders in nursing education and some leaders in nursing practice demand nurses prepared for leadership. These standards require nurses who are prepared to acquire advanced degrees, able to provide leadership for the profession, and able to exercise control over nursing practice.[14]

Incompatible standards

The standards of quality coming from each of these groups are often not compatible. The university values are generally neither accepted nor understood by the consumer or the nurse within the community. The expectations of the consumer and the community cannot be realistically met if the dean sets priorities based on the expectations of the university and on those of the nursing profession.

This conflict is compounded by related forces that may define the quality of nursing programs differently, for example, legal bodies such as boards of regents and state boards of nursing, federal agencies that affect funding, and associations of accreditation, resulting effectively in a "divide and conquer" syndrome—all lead deans into a maze of confusion, demanding a fine, balancing act. The end result for deans of nursing is one that is beneficial to other controlling bodies. They have effectively divided the profession.

The magic ingredient of "quality" that provides a measure of the success of the nursing program is elusive and unattainable and cannot be used to assist in providing justification for controlling our personal and professional destiny. However, the ingredient of "quality" is an important, elusive measure of success that can be used to affect the dean's accountability and vulnerability.

Consciously selecting the definition of quality and the groups to which the program is accountable is a basic step in achieving control of the discipline of nursing. As McGriff has stated in speaking about effective leadership in nursing, "We must have the courage of our convictions. We cannot change our story according to the audience, rather we must tell it like it is—regardless of how unpopular and painful the truth may seem."[15(p59)] As deans of nursing demonstrate their accountability to students and to health care consumers, these deans will define the quality of their programs in terms of standards that will improve the state of the nursing profession and of the health care of the community. Then sources of vulnerability can be analyzed and possible support sources identified.

SOURCES OF VULNERABILITY

There are four major sources of vulnerability generated by primary accountability to students and to health care consumers. Alternative sources of support can be developed in relation to each source of vulnerability. The choices made by deans in developing support are critical for the further development of nursing.

The university's economic and political environment

Stanton made the following statement concerning the importance of politics and power in policymaking:

> Politics, power and risk-taking must be present if nursing is to make an impact on health care. Politics is defined as the art of influence and is a part of everyday life. Power begins with the individual and evolves as an influence in relationships between people. Risk-taking means taking deliberate action where the consequences or outcomes are uncertain.[16(p20)]

It is almost impossible to separate the economic and political forces that affect the administering of an academic unit. Politics involves the total complex of relations between humans in a society and generally guides the making of social policy. Decision making involved in the development of policy is heavily laden with the use of power by those who control the environment. One of the most essential ingredients of politics, especially within a university, is having the power to control the economics of the institution and the educational unit. Piercy, a novelist and poet (see her poem at the introduction of this article),[17] defines politics as the exercise of values in society[18]—being able to define what is good and what is bad, who deserves and who does not deserve the resources of society and the environment.

As Taylor noted in 1934, nursing education has an equal right to the resources of the university, yet nursing programs are often viewed by university administrators as creating an undue economic burden on the institution. A program cannot be perceived as being an economic burden and have a strong influence or ability to control the decision-making process within the university.[19] Although other programs such as music or computer science may actually be more expensive than nursing, nursing education is generally considered one of the most costly programs. That is usually perceived as a negative fact, although until recently the cost of medical education has been less frequently discussed as an economic burden and has been accepted as a high priority.

Nursing programs are often viewed by university administrators as creating an undue economic burden on the institution.

The economic and political dynamics affecting many nursing education programs today mirror almost precisely the recorded history of the early Nightingale School of Nursing. The alleged closing of these schools was for economic reasons, although evidence exists that the real problems had to do with autonomy and the desire of politically powerful groups to control nursing education. The image of economic weakness is a powerful and oppressive force, placing nursing in a vulnerable position with academic peers, and provides a significant weapon for waging the war of control. The challenge for nursing deans once the reality of economic game playing is consciously analyzed, is to find ways to alter the perception of nursing as an economic burden on the institution and to demonstrate economic sufficiency based on realistic budgeting. Even though deans are largely measured by their ability to "wheel and deal" in the world of economic politics within the university, their basic task is to select strategies that will offset the power of the economic weapons used against them.

Political game playing involved in the exercise of accountability requires that political support systems be developed. Because the dean is a middle manager, such support systems need to come from many diverse groups that frequently have different goals, values, and commitments. The nature of the present social structure within and outside the university creates tremendous ideological and practical gulfs between various groups and subgroups. The dean is placed between the demands of the university administration and the faculty. Within the educational unit dichotomies occur between different faculty interest groups, such as graduate versus undergraduate faculty, the doctorally prepared versus the master's prepared, and tenured faculty versus nontenured faculty. The dean cannot expect to be all things to all people; in fact, the extent to which the deans attempt to satisfy the whims and demands of subgroups and opposing interest groups, the more they reinforce the continued existence of a "divide and conquer" syndrome. Decision making within such a context creates "wins" and "losses" among political supporters and leads to unhealthy conflict. This type of conflict can immobilize a group, negating progress toward any unified goal.

Given the assumption that nursing is a relatively oppressed group within the university, the dean's major challenge is to inspire unity in the faculty group. Subgroups will continue to exist, and there will be individual differences and disagreements. However, to the extent that the dean and the nursing faculty agree on the basic commitment to maintain the integrity of the profession and can perceive the reality of oppressive forces undermining this goal, the group can move together to overcome such forces in a healthy manner. Conflict among the faculty groups can be used as a means of perceiving the contradictions inherent in the situation and of identifying and selecting problem-solving approaches.[11]

Deans ultimately increase their strength to the extent that they consciously and deliberately decide how to use their energy and resources to gain and keep a political support system. However, to do so with the expectation of assuring personal survival as a dean is foolhardy. Potential and actual political support systems create difficult conflicts, disputes, and political struggles. Groups are often comprised of people overwhelmed by their own problems, apathetic and disinterested. Participants in groups move in and out in a fluid manner depending on their circumstances and motivation. Deans of nursing come and go regardless of the political networks of support developed from administrators and outside interest groups. The ultimate goal of a dean should center on what an individual's tenure as dean accomplished in achieving integrity and strength for the profession of nursing.

The relationship between nursing and power groups

Within the university and especially within a health sciences center, it is generally believed that the top administrations of the university and the medical community both in and outside the university have the greatest amount of power. Deans are often measured by their ability to collaborate effectively with these groups. *Collaboration* can mean to cooperate with or willingly assist an enemy in one's own country, especially an occupying force.[20] The thrust toward collaborating with medicine is contaminated with the reality that nurses are not generally viewed as peers or even as having a distinct profession by most physicians. Taylor stated in 1934 that schools of nursing and medicine must grow together but could not do so until nursing was free to develop the fundamental body of theory essential to the practice of the profession.[19] Today gains in this regard are encouraging, but nursing has not made sufficient gains in developing a body of knowledge to achieve a collegial relationship with medicine. As recently as 1965 the following perception of nurses by physicians was published in the *Journal of Medical Education:* "She must feel like a girl, act like a lady, think like a man and work like a dog."[21(p767)]

In the face of both historic and current evidence, one cannot deny the dominance of nursing by medicine. The underlying reasons for the dominance of nursing by medicine may be related to deeply rooted philosophic differences between the two disciplines, a relative lack of sophistication on the part of nursing in dealing with the academic and political requirements of the university and the health care system, or the fact that nurses are primarily women and physicians are primarily men. It is enlightening and helpful to understand and perceive accurately the underlying dynamics of this dominance, but the major obstacle for nurses to overcome is that of recognizing that this dominance is not a right and natural phenomenon. Consistent with the theory of oppression, nurses have been led to believe that it is right or natural for medicine to maintain control of the entire health care enterprise. The freedom to develop nursing's own destiny can only come from nursing's own initiative; it will not be freely granted by other groups.

Within a health science center dominated by physician administrators who control the standards of nursing education, achieving actual autonomy and accountability for nursing may be close to impossible and often depends on the personalities involved. One strategy that deans of nursing attempt to use is to gain the support of the highest level of administration in a university. However, this avenue is usually futile because of limited access or difficulty in communicating effectively about the inherent philosophical and practical contradictions between the disciplines of medicine and nursing.

Consistent with the theoretical framework of oppression, medical school deans and health science center administrators have significant advantages both in gaining access to and communicating with the highest level of a university administration. Nursing's lack of adequate data to analyze, support, and explain the nursing program's needs makes nursing deans appear less accountable and increases their vulnerability. Realistically, efforts need to be made in gaining the support of medical groups and of top level administration. However, a careful assessment of the potential for development of support from the groups is needed before taking a position and attempting to gain their support. Once a dean recognizes that a negative system or one that will yield nonsupport exists, data can be gathered related to their political and social power so as to be prepared both offensively and defensively when a power struggle emerges. The tendency of nursing deans to gain medicine's support at all costs leads deans to compromise the nursing profession, and accept token gains giving the illusion of autonomy and control of nursing education. The end result is an increase in their vulnerability to attack and control by medicine.

Women as deans

In describing the articles in the April 1980 issue of *Advances in Nursing Science* (2:3) dealing with the politics of care, the editor stated that

> It is critical to recognize the inherent relationship between the political problems of women and of nurses in today's culture. Although fewer than 2% of nurses are not women, well over 1.4 million nurses are women with political problems and challenges that are painful for any human to face, regardless of sex.[22(pxiv)]

Indeed, the problems that women deans face in male-centered universities are sufficient to drive the woman dean perfectly insane. An awareness of the reality of the dean's plight as a woman in universities is a giant step toward becoming "stark-raving sane." Denial of this fact does not contribute toward lessening the dean's vulnerability; denial only contributes to an increased vulnerability. The greatest vulnerability is blind acceptance of tokenisms that ultimately weaken the dean's accountability. Women scholars who have taken the plight of women in society seriously have begun to provide evidence that women tend to be basically powerless in terms of policymaking or influence as administrators. In a comparative analysis of governance within universities, faculty believed that deans have the broadest range of influence over decision making.[23] Inherent in this study is the fact that the majority of the deans involved were men and thus one cannot assume that women who were deans were perceived as having influence. Women who hold administrative or decision-making roles in academic institutions were documented as more likely than men to be unhappy and to have considerably less confidence in the top administrators of the institution than did their male colleagues.[23]

In the following statement Rich contrasted the current male-centered university with a potentially woman-centered university:

> Each woman in the university is defined by her relationship to the men in power instead of her

relationship with other women up and down the scale.... The structure of the man-centered university constantly reaffirms the use of women as a means to the end of male "work"—meaning male careers and professional success.[24(p137)]

Vance, in an analysis of women leaders, aptly described the overwhelming perceptual barriers (ie, distortions of reality) held by both men and women, particularly by women who attempt to achieve positions of power and influence in organizations:

It is my thesis that the woman who attempts to break out of the expected mold—who does not conform to the commonly accepted cultural feminine ideals and images—is often regarded as a *deviant*. Since in our society, professional leadership roles still typically fall within the male-assigned role, the woman who dares to be different—to be successful and exercise power in her own right—is a role breaker, an outsider. She fits into at least one or perhaps all of the definitions of deviance as conceptualized by Becker: varying too widely from the norm; something or someone essentially pathological; a symptom of social disorganization, and a failure to obey group rules.[25(p38)]

As women, nursing deans are vulnerable to being viewed with much the same sex stereotype as all other women in the university, including the majority of women employed by universities as secretaries, assistants, and clerks and literally functioning as a means to the end of male work. Because the deans' behavior often varies significantly from that of the stereotype, they are vulnerable to being viewed as deviant, to isolation from male power groups, and to isolation from other women in the university. Nursing deans are seldom appointed to prestigious and influential committees and are excluded from the most important decision-making groups. When women deans increase their influence and participation in decision making, they are vulnerable to a significant backlash. Diers proposed several axioms for nursing leadership, one of which speaks particularly to the problem of backlash and is consistent with the theoretical framework of oppression:

As women, nursing deans are vulnerable to being viewed with much the same sex stereotype as all other women in the university.

Paranoia gives one as clear and true a vision of the world as politics or religion.... what we are experiencing as nurses right now is backlash—an effect of the increasingly significant moves nursing is making both politically and in the delivery of services, and a reflection of the increasing power of women....

It is too easy to have one's nursing confidence undermined by backlash. But the other side of paranoia is to realize that we must be doing something right to be so important as to evoke these kinds of irrational responses. Backlash is a symptom of something else, and an implicit recognition that one's efforts have paid off.[26(p70)]

Dealing with the problems inherent in being a woman dean in a male-centered university creates a vicious cycle. The behaviors and actions that the dean might use to deal with this area of vulnerability increase her vulnerability because these behaviors are, by definition, role-breaking for the dean as a woman. Being a strong woman dean requires existential courage, "the courage to *see* and to *be* in the face of the nameless anxieties that surface when a woman begins to see through the masks of sexist society and to confront the horrifying fact of her own alienation from her authentic self."[27(p4)]

Solomon and Tierney, in a study of job satisfaction among college administrators, found that lower-level administrators were generally less satisfied with their jobs than were top-level administrators and that they made the best of the situation by setting limited and tangible goals.[28] Other mechanisms included recognizing strengths and weaknesses, laughing at oneself, seizing the opportunity to celebrate many occasions, and designating periods for reflective thought. The authors concluded that the best aid to general mental health is to find one's own rhythm or pattern of functioning that is productive and enhancing of one's sanity and depend on it for personal survival. Given the theoretical perspective of oppression, women in universities need not only recognize the problems of sexism in the university but also deliberately align themselves together as individuals and groups to begin to build a vital support system and overcome the divisions created by the existing social structure.

The dean as a person

The last source of vulnerability is perhaps the most important, that of the dean as a person. Vulnerability is perhaps most strongly influenced by the ability to maintain a sense of self-confidence. It is commonly assumed that the woman dean's personal life must be separated from the political and professional context in which she works and that emotions are irrelevant to the historical record created during one's tenure as a dean. Such an assumption and attempts to shape one's behavior based on it are unrealistic if the dean is to significantly contribute to the profession. The isolation created is one of the most powerful ways of undermining the dean's political strength, making the dean misunderstood and defenseless.

Cook, a contemporary historian who specializes in the study of women leaders of the nineteenth century and early twentieth century, has examined the relationship between the emotional support network and the political activism of women during that time period. In a recent article, she devoted a significant proportion of attention to the life and political impact of Lillian Wald, whom Cook recognizes to be one of the most significant women of her time period. Wald's personal support systems consisted of the long-term residents of Henry Street, including Annie Goodrich (who was involved in the loss of autonomy for nursing at Bellevue), Lavinia Dock, and other well-known nursing leaders of the time. Wald aligned herself with several affluent women who were involved in her work at the settlement and held close friendships with women who contributed financial support to her efforts. The records that Cook has examined indicate that these were not merely superficial friendships established for professional or political support; these women held strong emotional ties that nurtured and supported their professional and political successes.[29]

Deans frequently isolate themselves from the faculty on the assumption that the distance will facilitate objectivity in professional matters. Women deans also isolate themselves from the male-dominated higher administrative officers because any other way of relating may be viewed as inappropriate behavior having sexual overtones. Thus the female nursing dean typically hides behind her work, staying intensively active and supporting the rationalization that the inability to develop a satisfying personal support system is circumstantial.

Given the circumstances under which most nursing deans have developed personally and professionally in the existing social structure, it is predictable that the dean's behavior patterns in relation to the nursing faculty foster personal distance. A nursing faculty's struggle for freedom and their resistance to support a structure that dominates and inhibits optimum functioning create an environment in which the dean becomes the oppressor. Dominated and influenced by the ideologies and demands of the top-level administrator and other power groups, the dean tends to model her behavior after theirs, as Freire points out, to achieve privileges and power similar to those exhibited by the more powerful groups. Only when the dean discovers the reality of the situation in which she finds herself and begins to act in a humanizing way toward the faculty group will she begin to liberate herself and her coworkers.[11]

Consistent with the theory of oppression, leaders in nursing seem to hope for freedom while at the same time being afraid to attempt to achieve it. The fear can only be overcome by developing a support system, achieved through nurturing a sense of comradeship with peers, a willingness to give up the security of conformity, and a sense of who nurses need to be during the struggle for personal and professional identity. Confrontation with our own reality and expulsion of the myths that have been created and developed in the past can help transform a group, which in turn will free individuals within the group.[11] It is through a sense of unity and organization that the strength to recreate the world in which nurses live and work can be generated.

RESEARCH AND THEORY DEVELOPMENT

The theoretical framework of oppression has been used to analyze experiential observations made regarding the role and function of nursing deans in their efforts to establish accountability for nursing education and to identify the resulting vulnerabilities. Research is needed to verify these observations and interpretations, and to further develop theory that explains and predicts the social and political phenomena inherent in nursing education. The following specific research problems are suggested.

- What historical evidence exists regarding the social and political oppression of nursing as a health care discipline? What are the traits of nursing leaders who have historically contributed to the development of the discipline?
- What economic and political resources are actually available to nursing education programs in universities compared to other academic units? What are the processes by which the

distribution of resources is decided and what are the traits of individuals who tend to be the most influential in this process?

- On what basis is the "success" or "failure" of nursing deans judged, and do these criteria differ for different groups within the university and the community?
- What political support systems tend to be developed by nursing deans? What is the effect of the different sources of support on the nursing education program? Do these factors differ for deans in other disciplines?
- Are there different subjective responses or measurable outcomes to the same behaviors exhibited by men and women deans?
- On what model(s) do nursing deans base their political and social strategies? Do these differ from those of other academic deans or for male administrators?
- How do nursing faculty perceive and interpret nursing deans' behaviors? Which behaviors are perceived as enhancing the effectiveness of the group in achieving development personally and professionally?

REFERENCES

1. Nightingale F: *Cassandra* (with an introduction by Myra Stark and an epilogue by Cynthia Macdonald). Old Westbury, NY, Feminist Press, 1980. (Essay written in 1852)
2. Tooley SA: *The Life of Florence Nightingale.* New York, Macmillan Co, 1905.
3. Nightingale F: *Notes on Nursing: What It Is and What It Is Not.* New York, Dover Publications, 1969.
4. Kock HB: *Militant Angel.* New York, Macmillan Co, 1951.
5. Shryock R: *The History of Nursing: An Interpretation of the Social and Medical Factors Involved.* Philadelphia, WB Saunders, 1959 (an authorized facsimile by University Microfilm International, Ann Arbor, Mich).
6. Bruhn C: *Under the Authority of the Superintendent: An Autonomous Nursing School, Cincinnati, 1888–1896,* thesis. Wright State University, Dayton, Ohio, 1980.
7. Brown EL: *Nursing for the Future.* Philadelphia, Russell Sage Foundation, 1948.
8. Bridgewater SC: Organizational autonomy for nursing education. *J Nurs Educ* 18:4–8, January 1979.
9. Aydelotte M: Governance, education are watchwords for the 80's. *Am Nurse* 12:4, March 1980.
10. Ozimek D: *The Future of Nursing Education.* New York, National League for Nursing, 1975.
11. Freire P: *Pedagogy of the Oppressed.* New York, The Seabury Press, 1970.
12. Whittemore R: Faculty survival—Coping with managers. *Harper's,* February 1980, pp 38–41.
13. Hughes L: The public image of the nurse. *Adv Nurs Sc* 2:55–72, April 1980.
14. *Criteria for the Evaluation of Baccalaureate and Higher Degree Programs.* New York, National League for Nursing, 1977.
15. McGriff E: The courage for effective leadership in nursing. *Image* 8:56–60, October 1976.
16. Stanton M: Politics, risk-taking and nursing, in Williamson JA (ed): *Current Perspectives in Nursing Education: The Changing Scene.* St Louis, The CV Mosby Co, 1978, Vol II, pp 20–280.
17. Piercy M: The novel and the social process. Speech given at Wright State University, Dayton, Ohio, May 3, 1980.
18. Piercy M: The Low Road, in *The Moon Is Always Female.* New York, Alfred A. Knopf, 1980.
19. Taylor E: The rights of the school of nursing to the resources of the University. *Am J Nurs* 34:1187–1194, 1934.
20. *Webster's New Collegiate Dictionary.* Springfield, Mass, 1977.
21. Pratt H: The doctor's view of the changing nurse-physician relationship. *J Med Educ* 40:767–771, 1965.

22. Chinn PL: From the editor. *Adv Nurs Sci* 2:xiv, April 1980.
23. Baldridge V, Curtis D, Ecker G, Riley G: *Policy Making and Effective Leadership*. San Francisco, Jossey-Bass, 1978.
24. Rich A: *On Lies, Secrets and Silence*. New York, WW Norton, 1979.
25. Vance C: Women leaders: Modern-day heroines or societal deviants? *Image* 2:37–41, June 1979.
26. Diers D: Lessons on leadership. *Image* 2:67–71, 1979.
27. Daly M: *Beyond God the Father*. Boston, Beacon Press, 1973.
28. Solomon LC, Tierney ML: Determinants of job satisfaction among college administrators. *J Higher Educ* 48:412–431, 1977.
29. Cook BW: Female support networks and political activism: Lillian Wald, Crystal Eastman, Emma Goldman. *Chrysalis* 3:43–61, 1977.

Nursing Education, Professionalism, and Autonomy: Social Constraints and the Goldmark Report

Myrtle P. Matejski, M.S., M.A., Ph.D.
Assistant Dean and Associate Professor
College of Nursing
University of Rhode Island
Kingston, Rhode Island
Former Assistant Professor
School of Nursing
University of Maryland
Baltimore, Maryland

NURSING HAS BEEN DESCRIBED as a science and an autonomous discipline. However, it remains predominantly a women's profession. As such the professional autonomy of nurses is particularly vulnerable to the values of the society of which it is a part. One method of acquiring an appreciation of the interrelationship between societal attitudes and nursing progress is to study one segment in the evolution of modern secular nursing. Advances in science and technology, changes in medical education, altered social structure, cultural norms and values, and the political activity of women are all forces external to nursing that influence its autonomy. Each element merits an investigation of the interplay of social and internal factors as they have influenced the achievements of the profession. Only those elements that affect the client base of nursing will be addressed here. The selected factors that are described influenced the progress of nursing and nursing education immediately before and after the publication of the Goldmark report in 1923.

This article reflects the concepts of historical study exemplified by Holmes[1] and Butterfield.[2] Holmes indicated that the intensive study of a small situation provides a profitable way of understanding the historic development of a science.[1] Butterfield observed that case studies provide a means of visualizing "complicated movements that lie behind historic change."[2(p21)]

THEORETICAL FRAMEWORK

Sociological background

The nurse is a soldier. Absolute and unquestioning obedience is the fundamental idea of the military system.... Strictness and exactness produce better nurses.[3(p76)]

This quotation is attributed to Lavinia Dock in 1890. It indicates that the environment that fostered the nursing profession also encouraged an awe of authority, devotion to routine, and a retreat from initiative among nurses. Modern nursing educators may state that such subservience is fast receding. However, there still remain many areas in the United States where the attitude persists, nourished by nurses who resist change and supported by physicians and other social groups who still prefer to view women as dependents in a male-dominated society.

Clarke observed that general societal factors, attitudes, and economics are the inevitable, significant elements that are external to a profession and that shape its history.[4] For example, in the United States both medical education and nursing evolved in the nineteenth century during a period when the virtues of independence, competition, and free enterprise were extolled by philosophers, economists, educators, and politicians. Businessmen, craftsmen, and farmers were generally self-reliant and had no inclination to accept controls by governments or by regulating bodies.

Given the lack of constraints and the occasional need of individuals to receive nursing care, women who professed interest or special abilities in caring for the sick were able to become nurses. Among secular groups, formal vocational preparation for nursing was not available. There were few medical schools, so the majority of physicians and all nurses received their training as apprentices.[5]

Apprenticeship model

The advent in 1807 of the first successful proprietary medical school altered the apprenticeship methods of medical education. The prosperity enjoyed by the first proprietary venture soon encouraged the rapid development of similar institutions. No premedical education was required and the meager curriculum was frequently successfully completed in a few weeks.

Whereas apprenticeship methods included clinical practice, such experiences in the new schools were not only limited but were often nonexistent. Some schools offered clinical resources for an additional fee but if students could not afford to pay, they graduated without the clinical component.[6,7] This was in sharp contrast to nursing education which from its inception emphasized clinical practice. For both groups the pay was poor. Thus humane ideals and economic need provided the usual incentives for entrance into either field.[5] Further, the need to provide medical care to the citizens of a rapidly expanding nation encouraged the establishment of medical schools that could quickly produce physicians and encouraged interested women to nurse the sick. Thus social need and societal attitudes were influential in the development of both professions.

However, advances in science and technology required changes in medical education, if physicians were to provide adequate medical service. These advances also required changes in the kind of nursing care patients received. This meant formalizing the instruction for nurses. Fortunately for both medicine and nursing, the need to improve professional education in medicine and to establish professional training in nursing accompanied widespread reform movements in American society. As noted by Clarke, when conditions outside the profession became propitious, reform and change occurred.[4]

Baldridge noted that there are three major models of governance for organizations that can provide genuine insights into the functioning of organizations: bureaucratic, collegial, and political. The usefulness of each has been demonstrated in studies of academia. However, while each model can be useful in studies of professional organizations, Baldridge's political model as it relates to the profession of nursing is used in this report.

Political model

A political model is concerned with groups who can create pressure on the decision-making process of an institution or profession to promote change.[8] As is true with universities, professions are complex, pluralistic, social systems, with many groups pushing in various directions according to their special interests. As with universities, the pattern of interactions among the various groups shapes and reshapes the policies and decisions of the profession. Therefore the political model, which focuses essentially on description and explanation, provides a basis for understanding conflict, power, and decision making as these influence the autonomous nature of the group.

Many forms of pressure impinge on decision makers. Many studies have concerned internal conflicts among the various power blocs and interest groups within organizations. However, the least well-developed area in organizational theory relates to the influence of the external environment,[8] and it is this element that is addressed here.

Perceptive observers of the decision-making process are aware of the many external forces that impinge on professional organizations. Baldridge and Matejski observed that where professional organizations are well insulated from external pressures, the professionals themselves control the organization, determining its professional norms and defining its tasks and work routines.[8,9] Such organizations tend to possess a large measure of professional autonomy. However, where there is little insulation between an institution or professional organization and its environment, nonprofessional values can dominate it, resulting in a lessening of professional autonomy. Of particular concern to any professional group is its right and ability to determine its own membership. This right is manifested by the ability of the profession, for example, to control core tasks and decisions, such as determining admissions policies of applicants to the schools designed to prepare future professionals, to influence graduation criteria for students, and to affect the curriculum and goals of schools that educate future practitioners.

Other important elements of professional autonomy include the profession's ability to govern its affairs, to protect its members, to avoid nonprofessional control over professional work, and to establish and maintain its own internal organizational structure. All play important roles in the amount of autonomy a profession has. Each of these elements is, in turn, subject to three major sources of external pressure: financial dependency, clientele base, and direct environmental pressure.[8]

Financial dependency

Any organization or profession, if it is to survive and successfully achieve its mission, must have access to resources. Control over these resources (establishment of priorities and the allocation of funds) determines the course the organization or profession can follow. Therefore, the amount of external control an organization has over its funding will influence the amount of professional autonomy it enjoys. As explained by Baldridge and demonstrated by Matejski, when an organization becomes dependent on a limited source of funds, the contributors can exercise considerable influence on the expenditures of those funds, resulting in a decrease in the professional autonomy of the group.[8,9]

When an organization becomes dependent on a limited source of funds, the contributors can exercise considerable influence on the expenditures of those funds.

Clientele base

A second pressure is exerted by the particular clientele from which the professional group recruits its members. When the professional organization is confined to recruiting among persons with limited educational preparation, or where other restrictive factors, such as legal age requirements, sex, or religious preferences exist, or where a variety of occupational choices are available, the numbers of student nurses (clients) in the recruiting pool will be reduced. As a result the autonomy of the professional group will be limited.

Likewise where external factors influence the nature of the recruitment base (educational advantages, social class structure of potential clients), professional autonomy is lessened.[8] However, where there is access and appeal to a large, varied, well-prepared clientele, the profession can more easily implement its own standards, thus influencing its own progress toward its professional goals. Professional autonomy is thereby increased.[8]

Direct environmental pressure

Direct environmental pressure involves the deliberate imposing of values by groups external to the organization. For the nursing profession, medical groups, accreditation agencies, alumni, state boards of examiners, and state legislators are examples of external groups. The existence of persons or groups who offer values counter to those of the professional organization can have a significant effect. If, for example, there is a high concentration of interest groups in opposition to the goals of a profession, the profession itself may have difficulty withstanding the influence. This results in a low level of professional autonomy.

• • •

This article combines Clarke's theory that societal attitudes and economics shape the historical development of a profession with one major external source of pressure, client base, to describe and analyze specific problems that confronted nursing and nurse educators in the period following the Goldmark Report.

WOMEN, SOCIETY, AND ECONOMICS

The period following World War I was one of political conservatism: the emphasis of the political campaign of 1920 was on returning the country to "normalcy." Yet while the political attitudes of the electorate appeared to be conservative, society had experienced profound changes. The exposure of large numbers of Americans to European culture resulted in many of them returning to Europe as expatriates. World War I allowed middle-class American women to demonstrate their ability to assume a variety of roles in the work force. After the war many of them (approximately 24%) remained gainfully employed outside the home.[10] In addition, more middle-class women entered college than had attended before, and women had finally been granted the right to vote.

It is generally recognized that a healthy society has the ability to accept new kinds of uniformity and new ways of thinking. Thus the social changes in American society in the 1920s reflected the culmination of a period in the women's movement that extended from the mid-nineteenth century through the pre-World War I years. Feminists had increasingly urged that girls of every economic status become trained in some kind of income-producing career to fill up "vacant years" before marriage and to make women less vulnerable to potential economic catastrophes. The feminists were largely members of the upper middle class and had little real understanding of the life of middle-class women in America. Women who were not as well off financially as those in the middle classes and those who were less well educated tended to work in industry.[10]

The work ethic was strongly associated with the feminist idea of the role of women in society and as members of a work force. The work ethic was preached and taught by all religious groups. Leaders of the women's movement espoused the ethic particularly in terms of work outside the home. It was probably best expressed by Olive Shreiner and quoted in Rodgers:

> We demand that, in that strange new world that is arising alike upon the man and the woman, where nothing is as it was, and all things are assuming new shapes and relations. . . . we also shall have our own share of honored and socially useful human toil.[10(p182)]

The new ideas of a few people in one generation become the fashionable thoughts of the socioeconomic classes of the next and the common beliefs of the masses in the third.[11] Thus everyone is affected by what people of fashion considered important in an earlier generation. How quickly the change occurs is influenced by communication throughout the various levels of society.

The early feminists tended to be college-educated persons who recognized the social inequality of women. Women were victims of legal discrimination and nonentities in the ballot box. They were sexually exploited and medically misunderstood. Furthermore, when women worked outside the home, they were paid half a man's wages.[10] And because most feminists tended to view other women as women like themselves, bored with housework and underemployed, it is understandable that they saw what was wrong as a matter of women having lost their "productive work capacity."

However, during World War I women entered the work force and demonstrated their productive capability. Therefore feminists' views began to encroach on women in other social strata. The philosophical tenets of feminists and related social events affected society in general, and particularly women, during the decade of the 1920s. The ethic that dictated productive work for all segments of society also sanctioned the preparation of women for self-support as a hedge against financial need. The tendency to upward mobility through hard work encouraged women who toiled in factories to view nursing as suitable careers for their daughters, a career that could enable them to improve their social status and to achieve financial independence. It is against this background of political conservatism and social change that the Goldmark study was conducted.

The Goldmark study

The initial intent of the Goldmark study was to address the problems of public health nursing education. However, it soon became clear that the entire problem of nursing education needed to be studied. At the time of the study there were 1,755 schools of nursing in the United States, enrolling approximately 55,000 students, and graduating approximately 15,000 nurses per year.[12] Although the report addressed the financial dependency of the schools and the influence of outside agencies, this article focuses on the issue of the client base of the schools studied and the nature of the client problem generally as it influenced the nursing profession.

Following are some of the major recommendations of the Goldmark study:

- Reduction of the 3-year course to 28 months;
- Elimination of services of least value to the student, such as private duty and mending gloves;
- Radical reduction of other services to enable the students to concentrate efforts on educational pursuits;
- Elimination of monotonous repetition;
- Elimination of ward duty during the preliminary term;
- Ultimately demanding that entering students have a background in high school chemistry and dietetics;
- Completion of 4 years of high school as an admission requirement;
- Requirement that age of admission of

candidate coincide with age of graduation from high school;
- Replacement of student staff in hospitals with graduate nursing staff, thereby meeting the educational needs of students separately from patient needs; and
- Specialized hospitals or small hospitals unable to provide broad experiences for their student nurses abandoning the attempt of nursing education.[12]

All of these suggestions were reasonable, and nursing leaders tended to support the recommendations of the report. However, even though some nursing schools ultimately closed, there seems to have been no widespread change. Certainly the impact of the Goldmark report on nursing did not equate with the results of the Flexner report in medicine.

The Flexner report

Flexner's report, published in 1910, encouraged reforms in medical education that were virtually completed by all surviving medical schools by 1920. Yet as recently as 1964 some schools of nursing had yet to meet a majority of the recommendations of the 1923 Goldmark report. Why was there such a delay?

Merton suggested that social action is not taken until the public becomes aware of the violation of accepted norms.[13] The Flexner report was widely disseminated among medical educators and the news media, from the *New York Times* to the *El Paso* (Texas) *News*. Further, it provided the names of each institution visited, as well as the specific observations about the educational facilities available to the medical students. Such publicity affected students seeking medical education. In addition, leading practitioners and medical educators for years had sought reform in medical education, and the medical profession had long enjoyed considerable professional autonomy. These factors, combined with society's support for reform, provided an atmosphere conducive to the acceptance of change.

The Goldmark report, in contrast, although no less critical of nursing and nursing education, was considerably less influential in encouraging change. The report did not name specific institutions as representative of good or poor schools. Its findings were not widely published in the news media. Consequently, even though nursing leaders recognized the need for reform, the public remained generally uninformed about the needs for change. Further, there was no other widespread reform movement occurring elsewhere when the report was published.

Finally, nursing was not autonomous. Hospitals opened the schools of nursing, paid stipends to students to enroll, and were the agencies that determined which nursing clients should enter the profession and how they should be educated. In addition, the notion of women's roles and male dominance, so widely prevalent, did little to encourage or support the call for change.

There were other reasons for the apparent nonacceptance of the recommendations of the report. The science of nursing depends on the mobilization of relevant knowledge from a number of disciplines and also on cultural and social changes. Like medicine, it is rooted in the culture and practical needs of the society it serves. Unlike the period of reform prior to and following the Flexner report, the period of

Employing nurses in army hospitals only relieved men of tasks that would not have been entrusted to nurses under peacetime conditions.

the Goldmark report reflected conflicting philosophies between political and social norms, between a political emphasis on conservatism and a return to the past, and societal elements that were attempting to change direction. Because of war, many women became useful in a variety of fields and nurses demonstrated their abilities to serve responsibly in the health care field.

Such incursions, however, were viewed as appropriate only for a short time. Employing nurses in army hospitals only relieved men of tasks that would not have been entrusted to nurses under peacetime conditions because society still considered men to be rulers. Physicians were still considered leaders of the health team, governing all matters related to health, illness, and the education of the team members.

PHYSICIAN CONTROL OVER THE CLIENT BASE

Who would provide care for patients was of prime concern for physicians. Hospitals were concerned with how to provide adequate care at the least cost. Both factors played a significant role in supporting the apprenticeship type of education that physicians had long since abandoned. Both concerns were reflected in physician and hospital attitudes about nursing education and its potential influence on medical practice and medical education. One example can be found in the 1920 *Bulletin of the University of Maryland School of Medicine and College of Physicians and Surgeons:* "The shortage of student nurses has become so acute at this institution that it threatens to seriously handicap the instruction of students of the medical school."[14(p107)] As for the need for nursing students to provide cheap service, there can be no doubt: ". . . it is impossible to secure graduates to do the work, even if we were financially able to pay the salary demanded."[14(p108)]

The bulletin noted that if physicians were unable to attract desirable women to enter "our Training School," the work of the hospital would have to be curtailed. This, of course, would be detrimental to a medical school that was struggling to meet the criteria required for its own accreditation. The word *desirable* is not defined, although evidence supports the notion that there was concern for attracting women from at least middle-class families.

SOCIAL AND ECONOMIC FACTORS AND THE CLIENT BASE

The decline in the numbers of "desirable women" entering nursing in the 1920s appears to have been a reflection of increased opportunities for women in other occupations. Thus the client base began to change. Women whose families could afford it attended college, thereby markedly reducing the numbers of women in the higher and middle socioeconomic groups who entered nursing.[12] Thus the 1927 Burgess report shows that a larger number of nurses than would normally be expected came from families of foreign-

born parents who tended to be employed in factories.[15]

In nursing, as in the rest of American society, the work ethic was strongly in force. Long hours, difficult and menial chores, little time away from the duties of the hospital, and public acceptance of these policies all attest to the widely prevalent belief in hard work. The goal was to become independent by working hard. For families in the lower socioeconomic brackets, the admission of a daughter to a school of nursing that enabled her to become a registered nurse was evidence that hard work had results.

As difficult as nursing was, the work appeared to be less hard and tedious than factory labor. Nursing was a socially acceptable means of support for women until they married, and it was a hedge against potential economic difficulties. The significance of the work ethic in America helps explain why parents and students offered little criticism of the apprentice-type education that persisted in nursing. As might be suspected, daughters of lower socioeconomic classes migrated readily to nursing. However, during the 1920s there were many nursing schools, and daughters of "good" families could be highly selective in their choices.[15] As a result, just as proprietary medical schools had accepted students with questionable educational background, so too the smaller, more service-oriented schools of nursing tended to attract young women with inferior educational backgrounds. Thus in 1927, 11% of hospital staff nurses and 20% of "floating" nurses had an eighth-grade education or less, and only 34% of the staff nurses included in the Burgess study had 4 years of high school education.[15]

EDUCATIONAL PREPARATION AND THE CLIENTS

Baldridge observed that where there is a large, well-prepared recruiting pool, a profession can more easily implement its own admission standards and school requirements, thereby improving the autonomy of both the schools and the profession. However, in nursing professional autonomy remained low. However much nursing leaders in the 1920s may have wished to establish higher standards of admission for nursing students, schools dependent on hospitals for support were rarely in a position to improve admissions requirements.

As a result educational boards, comprised largely of hospital and physician representatives, impeded improvements in nursing education. This is readily demonstrated in Maryland where, for example, minutes of the University of Maryland Medical School faculty reveal considerable discussion concerning the expulsion of several student nurses because of their academic or clinical performance and question the authority of the nursing superintendent to make such a decision.[16]

Admission requirements

Statistical data from the Goldmark study also support the Baldridge thesis that an important relationship exists between the client base from which a profession can recruit and professional autonomy. Of the 23 schools of nursing the commissioners reviewed, 13 required 4 years of high school, 3 required 2 years of high school, 6 required 1 year of high school, and 1 reported that it tried to meet state requirements for 1 year of high school.[12] Of the schools included in the Goldmark study, approximately 22% of the students had not graduated from high school. Most nursing school catalogues indicate only that such preparation was desirable, again reflecting the influence of clients on the autonomy of schools of nursing.

The 1925-1926 catalogue of the University of Maryland School of Nursing (a diploma program at the time) stated that applicants to the school were expected to show evidence of a high school education or its equivalent. No mention is made of how much high school education is required, nor what subjects ought to be included as preparatory to nursing.[17] Evidence of the equivalence of courses to high school courses consists of a written statement by the high school principal.

The Mercy Hospital Training School for Nurses also required a high school education or its equivalent. Maryland General Hospital Training School added a statement that applicants had to pass an examination in subjects "embraced in or equivalent to four years' curriculum in high schools of the state of Maryland."[17(p102)] This then suggests that although 4 years of high school education was desirable, other factors precluded making it a requirement.

Documents reveal that had such education been available, there is no certainty that the large percentage of female students would have had either the opportunity to attend high school or that the curriculum offered would have prepared them for the subject matter encountered in nurses' training programs. Again Maryland exemplifies the kind of educational problems experienced by many women living in other parts of the country.

In 1921 Flexner, in a report concerning state-aided colleges in Maryland, noted that there were only 1,626 girls graduating yearly from public and private high schools combined.[18(p16)] Of the total number of high school graduates of both sexes (2,512), only 25% were enrolled in college. At the time of Flexner's study Maryland had three women's colleges, four coeducational institutions, and three normal schools or teachers' colleges. In addition, women were admitted to the various departments of the University of Maryland such as education, home economics, pharmacy, and the School of Medicine. There were also 19 schools of nursing in Baltimore City plus 6 in the counties. The client base for nursing was clearly limited, and the situation did not improve greatly during the decade of the 1920s.

By 1930 there were 4,320 white women and 636 black women between the ages of 18 and 19 attending school. The statistics are not clear as to the level of education that is represented here, but glancing at the numbers of women aged 20-21 who were still receiving education in succeeding years, it would appear that roughly one-third of the 18 to 19-year-old women were involved in post-high-school study (Table 1).[19] In the meantime, the numbers of occupations open to women had increased. There were more schools, and the numbers of diploma schools of nursing had grown to 31, along with three practical nursing programs.[20]

Educational differences

This situation demonstrates the problem schools of nursing experienced in recruiting high school graduates. With large

Table 1. Population attending school

Population attending school (ages 15–20)	White males	White females	Black males	Black females
Urban—1920	10,029 (27%)	8,388 (22.4%)	1,020 (18.8%)	1,427 (19.8%)
Rural—1920	7,732 (29%)	7,517 (32%)	1,958 (24%)	1,931 (27%)
Urban—1930	16,044 (39%)	14,060 (33.4%)	1,838 (26.7%)	2,415 (27%)
Rural—1930	10,683 (34%)	10,546 (38%)	1,645 (20%)	1,576 (23%)
Population attending school—1930 (ages 18-19)				
Total	5,342 (22%)	4,320 (18.9%)	412 (8%)	636 (11.7%)

numbers of schools from which to choose, better prepared students had a variety of options. Thus although the Goldmark report declared that students with only 2 years of high school education lacked the background necessary for understanding the subject matter essential to professional nursing training, many schools were unable to compete for better students. Moreover, schools' need for financial support and the hospitals' desires for low-cost patient services encouraged schools of nursing to compete for students by paying stipends and providing school uniforms, books, living quarters, and meals in return for apprentice training. Furthermore, as physicians moved to admit larger numbers of patients to hospitals, the demands for service increased, putting even more pressures on schools of nursing to enlarge their enrollments. The limited pool of qualified applicants, in the face of all the aforementioned conditions, contributed to a low professional autonomy for nurses and the schools in which they taught.

The limited pool of qualified applicants . . . contributed to a low professional autonomy for nurses and the schools in which they taught.

Nor were these the only educational problems facing women who wished to pursue careers in medicine or nursing. Herriott and Hodgkins indicated that the "degree of modernity of an educational system varies as a function of the degree of modernity of its sociocultural environment."[21(p16)] Evidence shows that the high school education provided frequently differed for boys and girls and among schools in urban and rural areas. In Maryland for instance urban schools might have students spend more time studying science and the humanities, but rural schools tended to prepare students for life in rural settings. Consequently the curriculum for girls was more likely to concentrate on home economics and the kinds of information perceived by a rural society as "practical."[22] As a result the rural areas of Maryland were an unproductive source of students for colleges in general because the high school curriculum did not include the subjects required for college admission.[22] Even where female students had graduated from high school, there was little to suggest that the subjects they took would prepare them for the courses the Goldmark study proclaimed necessary. Courses such as chemistry or biology were frequently not included. Thus there was a limited number of adequately prepared potential nursing students relative to the numbers necessary to support the hospitals and their nursing programs financially. This situation was no doubt repeated in rural areas and small towns throughout the country. In an attempt to assure sufficient numbers of students to provide patient care, hospital schools of nursing admitted probationers three, four, and sometimes up to six times per year.[12,14,17] The admissions standards were essentially dictated by local school systems and social attitudes.

Nursing, despite its struggle to achieve true professional status and autonomy, was caught in the dilemma of social attitudes about education for women, the opening of new occupations to women, the expanding technology of medical practice that encouraged hospitalization of patients, the need of hospitals to provide inexpensive patient services, and the work ethic. Faced with these problems, nursing did well to survive and to achieve a measure of autonomy and professional status.

AN EXPANDED PERSPECTIVE

One purpose of this article is to introduce nursing historians to a somewhat different approach to the study of nursing history, using a theoretical framework that views the problems of professionalism and its constraints in terms of social norms, financial dependence, clientele base, and direct environmental pressures. Using this framework the problems confronting women generally, the work ethic, and the relationship of the whole to the problems confronting nursing education during the 1920s have been addressed. An effort has been made throughout this article to describe and explain the issue of the clientele base of nursing as an element important to the understanding of where nursing has been as a profession, why it occupied its position in the decade of the 1920s, and some of the variables that must be considered in viewing nursing progress.

Parsons and Platt have noted that when universities became the main locus of scientific study, forward-looking medical educators demanded that physicians be educated where the applications of science and technology could be demonstrated clinically.[23] Thus the competence of applied professions relies on their effective use of basic research in clinical practice. Only a few nursing leaders in 1923 recognized this truism for nursing, but over time nursing education has assumed its appropriate position in academia. Considering the obstacles American nursing had to overcome, nursing ought not to be apologetic about having taken a while to achieve professional status.

Faced with the complexities of medical practice, nurses have often been placed in positions of assuming functions formerly reserved for physicians but without having the formal preparation to assure more than intuitive actions. Based on the Goldmark and Burgess studies, nursing instituted reform although not to the extent needed. Insufficiently prepared client bases as well as lack of financial support contributed to the slow progress made. To realize the extent of nursing's progress and to assure its continued growth, it is important for nursing historians to document the nature of past constraints to nursing education and professionalism, to assess the profession against the background of society in general, and to be alert to potential similar problems in the future.

For those who would administer schools of nursing with the greatest amount of autonomy, the message is clear. Schools of nursing of necessity must establish curricula that will appeal to the broadest numbers of clientele. In some cases this means upgrading requirements for admission of candidates at all levels; in particular it means establishing a curriculum that reflects clearly stated goals of producing nursing leaders.

This also means acknowledging the need to prepare professional nurse practitioners at all levels in yet greater depth and breadth than is currently being done. And it means inculcating into neophytes their responsibilities in communicating needs and goals to all segments of society. As noted by Baldridge[8] and documented by Matejski[9], when the client base becomes extended so as to attract students from beyond the local environment, autonomy of the profession and the school improves. This provides an added dividend. As the graduates of a program become known for their work, quality, and research, more students with similar potentials are attracted to the school. As more of the school's graduates move into positions of leadership, financial support from alumni increases, providing more autonomy for the profession and its schools. Each element improves the whole.

As the problems of nursing education in the 1920s are reviewed, it seems clear that had nursing leaders been more communicative with educators in secondary schools and with the public, needed changes in nursing education conceivably could have been achieved earlier. It is also clear that nursing faces many similar problems today. Nurses need to be cognizant of their past and to learn whatever lessons they may from it. Above all nurses need to become acutely aware of the variety of societal factors that can impede their progress and to learn how to advance in the face of social and economic constraints.

The canvas of nursing history here has been painted with broad brush strokes, but an attempt was made from time to time to illustrate fine figures through detailing specific problems within one small state. Much more detail must be included to assure a full understanding of the evolution of nursing.

> Human affairs being the subject matter of history, all human pursuits and disciplines in their social aspects enter into it. But as no human mind can master more than a fraction of what would be required for a wide and balanced understanding of human affairs, limitation and selection are essential to the historian's craft.[24]

REFERENCES

1. Holmes FL: The case study method in the historiography of medical sciences, in *Modern Methods in the History of Medicine*. London, The Athlone Press, 1971.

2. Butterfield N: *The Whig Interpretation of History.* London, G Bell, 1951.
3. Johns E, Pfefferkorn B: *The Johns Hopkins Hospital School of Nursing 1889–1949.* Baltimore, Johns Hopkins University Press, 1954.
4. Clarke EC (ed): *Modern Methods in the History of Medicine.* London, The Athelone Press, 1971.
5. Shryock RH: Nursing emerges as a profession: The American experience, in Leavitt JW, Numbers RL (eds): *Sickness and Health in America.* Madison, Wisc, The University of Wisconsin Press, 1973.
6. Woodworth JR: Some influences on the reforms in schools of law and medicine 1898-1930. *Sociol Quart* 14:96, 1973.
7. Duffy J: *The Healers: A History of American Medicine.* Chicago, University of Chicago Press, 1976.
8. Baldridge JV: Introduction. Models of university governance—bureaucratic, collegial, and political, in Baldridge JV (ed): *Academic Governance: Research on Institutional Politics and Decision-Making.* Berkeley, Calif, McCutcheon Publishing Corp, 1971.
9. Matejski MP: The influence of selected external forces on medical education at the University of Maryland School of Medicine, 1910-1950, dissertation. University of Maryland, Baltimore, 1977.
10. Rodgers DT: *The Work Ethic in Industrial America, 1850–1920.* Chicago, University of Chicago Press, 1978.
11. Barzun J: Cultural history as synthesis, in Stern F (ed): *The Varieties of History from Voltaire to the Present.* New York, World Publishing Co, 1956.
12. Goldmark J: *Nursing and Nursing Education in the United States, Commission for the Study of Nursing Education.* New York, Macmillan Co, 1923.
13. Merton RK: *The Student Physician: Introducing Studies in the Sociology of Medical Education.* Cambridge, Mass, Harvard University Press, 1969.
14. *Bulletin of the University of Maryland School of Medicine and College of Physicians and Surgeons* 5:107, 1920.
15. Burgess MA: *Nurses, Patients and Pocketbooks: A Report of a Study on the Economics of Nursing.* New York, Committee on the Grading of Nursing Schools, 1928.
16. University of Maryland Medical School, Minutes of the Faculty of Physics, May 8, 1918.
17. *Bulletin of the University of Maryland School of Medicine and College of Physicians and Surgeons,* vol 22, 1925.
18. Flexner A: *Report of General Education Board—State-Aided College in Maryland, to the Governor of Maryland,* 1921.
19. *16th Census, Maryland II, 1940: Population, Second Series, Characteristics of the Population of Maryland.* US Bureau of the Census, 1942.
20. *Twenty-Fifth Anniversary of the Maryland State Nurses' Association: An Historical Sketch 1903–1928.* Baltimore, JH Furst Co, 1928.
21. Herriott R, Hodgkins B: *The Environment of Schooling: Formal Education as an Open Social System.* Englewood Cliffs, NJ, Prentice-Hall, 1973.
22. *Report of the State Board of Education.* Maryland House and Senate Documents, 1911, pp 77-127.
23. Parsons T, Platt GM: *The American University.* Cambridge, Mass, Harvard University Press, 1973.
24. Namier L: History and political culture, in Stern F (ed): *The Varieties of History from Voltaire to the Present.* New York, World Publishing Co, 1956.

The Administrative Component of the Nurse Administrator's Role

Margaret L. McClure, R.N., Ed.D., F.A.A.N.
Director of Nursing
Maimonides Medical Center
Brooklyn, New York

THE ADMINISTRATIVE components of the nurse administrator role are difficult to analyze for two reasons: on the one hand, they appear to be too obvious to warrant discussion; on the other hand, they appear to be too global in scope for meaningful exploration in a brief article. Therefore, rather than focus on all the administrative aspects of the nurse administrator's role, it is more useful to highlight only those that are unique. With this as a foundation, the question as to how one might prepare nurses to become administrators can then be addressed.

UNIQUE PROPERTIES OF THE NURSE ADMINISTRATOR'S ROLE

On close examination, it becomes obvious that the unique properties of

This article is based on a presentation at the "Nursing Administration: Directions for the Future" invitational conference sponsored by the Boston University School of Nursing, November 3 and 4, 1978.

the nurse administrator's role are not so much unique in and of themselves as they are unique in the particular combinations in which they present themselves. These properties may be classified into four broad categories:

1. the nature of the work;
2. the nature of the workers;
3. the nature of the internal environment; and
4. the nature of the external environment.

Nature of the Work

TWENTY-FOUR HOUR RESPONSIBILITY

The department of nursing, like many other service-oriented departments, is highly labor intensive; in addition, it has the responsibility in inpatient settings for providing continual service on a 24-hour basis, every day. While other occupations may lay claim to similar obligations to their clients, it would seem that nursing is singular among the *professions* in this regard. In fact, recently a physician raised the question as to whether the 24-hour nature of much of nursing's work might not be responsible for its difficulty in gaining recognition as a full-fledged profession. The physician cited the need for constant on-duty, rather than simply on-call personnel as a deterrent to the image of the autonomous professional since such demands result in "shift" work. Such a hypothesis underscores the uniqueness of nursing's 24-hour responsibility.

Clearly this 24-hour responsibility carries with it a large number of interrelated and difficult administrative problems. For example, how does one attract and retain qualified nursing staff to work during those hours when the majority of other professionals and nonprofessionals are not working? Underlying this is a larger question: how does one maintain acceptable and consistent standards of patient care around the clock? There are still other questions. For instance, how does one provide educational opportunities, related directly or indirectly to nursing care, for the entire staff? How can changes in policy be effectively communicated to all the staff, keeping in mind that it is never possible to schedule a single meeting that all may attend? This small sample of questions touches only superficially on the kinds of problems that arise from the 24-hour responsibility. They are, however, representative of an array of administrative concerns with which the nurse administrator must deal.

LACK OF ABILITY TO PREDICT AND/OR CONTROL WORK FLOW

A second important characteristic related to the administration of nursing is the difficulty encountered in predicting and/or controlling the work flow. Thompson has observed that organizations as a whole will attempt to gain control of their work flow in order to survive.[1] He describes a number of means by which this control may be accomplished, the least satisfactory of which is rationing of scarce resources. An organized nursing service, however, is hard pressed to utilize, to any great extent, any mechanisms that might assist in the rationalization of the work flow problem, although in certain situations rationing has met with limited success.

There are three important variables that influence the work flow for nursing. These are (1) problems of patients and their families, (2) advances in medical technology and (3) changes in philosophy and/or funding.

Certainly the fact that unpredictable problems often arise for patients and their families comes as no surprise to any nurse. To a certain extent, it is this very characteristic that attracts many to the profession and keeps them interested in it. The emergency craniotomy performed at 2:00 A.M., the sudden call for the cardiopulmonary resuscitation team on an otherwise quiet Sunday afternoon, the school bus accident resulting in the arrival of ten injured children—all of these are relatively frequent occurrences that cannot be predicted but nonetheless have enormous impact on nursing's workload. Administering a department that is prepared to cope with such crises while continuing to maintain care for the predicted and so-called routine patient needs is no small task.

Administering a department that is prepared to cope with such crises while continuing to maintain care for the predicted and so-called routine patient needs is no small task.

The second variable, that of advances in medical technology, is less dramatic in its impact on the nursing workload; however, it is also more problematic in that it tends to be gradual and incremental in nature and thus more difficult to document. For example, within the past decade alone, cardiac monitoring, pressure respirators and hyperalimentation therapy have become increasingly commonplace outside of intensive care settings. The insidiousness of these advances, however, makes the resultant input overload for nursing difficult to address.

The third variable, changes in philosophy and funding, is closely related to the problem of advances in medical technology. Probably the most publicized instance of this type of change is in the area of end-stage renal disease. In recent years, the liberal federal funding for these patients has led to enormous increases in the use of hemodialysis and peritoneal dialysis. Individuals, who only a few years ago would have been denied access to such therapies, are now routine recipients and create a demand for nurses skilled in their care. While the merits of the program can probably not be argued, the effect on the nursing workload remains an issue.

In dealing with the variables related to work flow, the nurse administrator must not only be cognizant of their impact but also be prepared to analyze them. There is little question that the development of patient classification tools offers an important aid in this regard. Further development and refinement will undoubtedly increase their value in years to come. It should be kept in mind, however, that in a world of scarce resources, sound analysis of a problem does not ensure that the means for solving the problem will necessarily follow.

PHYSICAL ASPECTS OF THE WORK

Another administrative property that is related to the nature of nursing is the physical aspect of the work. This dimension is rarely discussed today, although in reality it has not decreased to any degree and has probably increased in many settings. Perhaps the emphasis that has been placed on the intellectual aspects of nursing in recent years has caused the physical component to be underplayed. The fact remains that the physical demands of the job are such that "burnout" is becoming more commonplace among staff nurses, and concern for this phenomenon is mounting.

Added to the problem of the "burnout" syndrome among relatively young nurses is the question of appropriate placement of staff who are no longer young or who become disabled. In most acute care settings, the number of positions that might be offered to such individuals has decreased as the acuity of illness of patients has increased. Simply stated, it is becoming more and more difficult to grow old in the profession of nursing.

The fact remains that the physical demands of the job are such that "burnout" is becoming more commonplace among staff nurses, and concern for this phenomenon is mounting.

Again, while it is true that many other occupations deal with work that is physically demanding, nursing is somewhat unique in this regard among the *professions.* The nurse administrator is often hard pressed to support and meet the needs of the staff while at the same time ensuring that patients' physical needs are adequately met.

The Nature of the Workers

THE MIX OF PROFESSIONAL AND NONPROFESSIONAL WORKERS

Nursing care is generally delivered in most settings by a mixture of professional and nonprofessional workers. In this regard, it is probably not very different from other occupations, although the numbers of levels and categories may be somewhat unique. What is, of course, truly peculiar to nursing is the diversity of preparation and ability within the group designated as "professional." No other field of endeavor issues professional licenses to individuals educated at such a variety of levels. What is of interest here is the problem that such diversity creates for the administrator. These basically fall into two categories, one being professional practice and the other being employee behaviors.

As far as professional practice is concerned, the director of nursing often finds that the staff lacks the degree of knowledge and skill required to meet particular patient needs, in spite of the fact that there are large numbers of so-called professionals among them. Furthermore, in many situations there are sets of variables operating that may preclude the recruitment of persons with the appropriate knowledge levels. Geographic location, safety of the neighborhood, reputation of the hospital and the type of patient the hospital cares for are some of the factors that affect prospective staff. Clearly this problem impacts on every practice issue with which the director must deal, whether it be quality assurance programs, joint practice committees or interagency referrals. Without a substantial cadre of knowledgeable staff, the director is stymied in every effort to move clinical practice forward.

Without a substantial cadre of knowledgeable staff, the director is stymied in every effort to move clinical practice forward.

In the area of employee behaviors, the impact of the diversity is more subtle, yet it has some very real complicating ramifications. For example, it is impossible to expect professional norms and values to operate in regard to such matters as self-governance and individual accountability when there are distinct differences among the persons involved. For the administrator, an approach to the group must be achieved that will not overextend what is attainable by some, but will, by the same token, meet the needs for self-direction and autonomy that the more professional staff members might have. Dealing with the registered nurse group as if they were all true professionals is likely to be as unsuccessful as dealing with them as if they were all nonprofessionals would be.

A FEMALE PROFESSION

A second property that cannot be overlooked in a discussion of the nature of the workers is the fact that the field is composed predominantly of women. Because of this, almost every individual practicing within the occupation is simultaneously engaged in the dual careers of nurse and homemaker. The ramifications of this dual role playing are great and should not be minimized; they touch every aspect of employment.

At the outset, recruiting women is different from recruiting men for similar positions. For example, women who work and have household responsibilities at the same time cannot afford to commute long distances. Furthermore, relocation of a married female worker depends, more often than not, on the husband's job situation. Unfortunately for nursing it is still rare to hear of a man deciding to relocate because his wife received an important job offer in a different geographic area. Thus recruitment techniques that are successful for other fields do not readily apply to nursing.

Once the female nurse accepts a position, shift rotation and weekend and holiday work become issues of concern. Obviously, this problem relates directly to the question regarding nursing's 24-hour responsibility. The fact is that nurses must be available to care for patients, regardless of how unpopular the hour. Significant others tend to have little sympathy with this situation. There is, of course, an interesting cultural double standard operating here. The female school teacher who is married to a male police officer *expects* to rearrange the family's life to accommodate her husband's shift rotation. In fact, all of society expects this. However, in spite of important gains made by the women's movement, we have not yet arrived at the point where the male accountant married to the female nurse *expects* to rearrange the family's life to accommodate his wife's shift rotation.

We have not yet arrived at the point where the male accountant married to the female nurse ex-* pects *to rearrange the family's life to accommodate his wife's shift rotation.

Another problem related to female role-taking behavior is that nurses tend to be quite passive as a group. Kinsella recently observed that there are "an increasing number of nurses for whom the norm is independent, assertive behavior."[2] While one might agree to some extent that the number of such individuals is increasing, there are certainly too few of them to date; and this has a serious impact for any practice setting in which an administrator is attempting to upgrade the nursing care delivered to patients. Too many within the profession tend to be passive rather than active.

> To be more specific, nurses seem to be psychologically geared to *respond* to others rather than to initiate action. The physician writes an order, the nurse carries it out. The patient rings his bell, the nurse answers it. Perhaps because of this fairly typical sequence of events, nurses have developed a patterned approach to patient care that is almost akin to a conditioned response. This set of circumstances creates problems with which we have been attempting to deal for many years.[3]

Unfortunately there is evidence that passivity is a function of female sex role identity,[4] although there is also ample evidence that such behavior patterns can be altered if the proper circumstances are provided.[5] The task for the nurse administrator is to convince the staff that the verb "to nurse" need not be operationalized only in the passive voice.

A final ramification of the nursing work force being predominantly female is the fact that the dual role of homemaker and nurse often results in interrupted career patterns for nursing. In industry, white collar workers are frequently placed in long-term training programs—some as long as five years—for the express purpose of developing a highly professional work force.[6] This is a luxury that a predominantly female occupation cannot enjoy. Indeed, a fairly substantial proportion of nursing turnover in any health care facility is related to such domestic responsibilities as child rearing or family relocation due to the demands of the husband's occupation.[7] Nurses characteristically enter and leave the field in patterns that are both expected and predictable.

This creates obvious problems for the nurse administrator, not only in terms of recruitment and orientation, but more importantly in the provision of continuity for program development. All innovations must be designed in such a way that substitutions of key personnel can be accomplished with ease and without a great deal of notice. Clearly, the more specialized we become, the more difficult this is to achieve.

Nature of the Internal Environment

THE POWER OF THE PHYSICIAN

Probably one of the most commonly accepted properties of the internal environment of health care facilities is the all-pervasive power of physicians, in spite of the fact that they are to all intents and purposes, visitors to the institution in the majority of cases. To a large extent, physician power is a splendid example of the facetious golden rule in action: the fellow with the gold makes the rules. In the past, this problem has been discussed with a seeming air of mystery surrounding it, in a manner somewhat akin to the "blue smoke and mirror" phenomenon that Jimmy Breslin describes when he discusses political power.[8] In fact, there is nothing mysterious about physician power; it is merely a function of economics. The physician and only the physician can bring in the customers. Given the precarious financial situations in most health care agencies today, the customer is the key to survival. Empty beds are the forerunners of bankruptcy, a fearful reality with which many hospitals have been forced to deal in the decade of the seventies.

Thus physicians must be catered to and courted, and the more options they have open to them in regard to institutions in which they may hospitalize their patients, the more power they are likely to have. This creates problems for directors of nursing only insofar as they generate opposition from a physician or physicians as a result of some program they are involved in or as a result of personal animus. The consequences of such opposition can be quite serious, even devastating, for the director.

INTERDEPENDENCE OF MEDICINE AND NURSING

Another property related to the internal environment that has been tacitly understood but has probably received too little attention is nursing's unique relationship with medicine. The interdependence between the two affects the work and the outcomes of both to a high degree. Each affects the quality of the other; thus neither can achieve a degree of excellence without the other. This is demonstrated repeatedly in hospital settings and is the cause of a great deal of tension between the two.

A patient who is admitted to a hospital for a mitral valve replacement may have the most competent and knowledgeable surgeon in the nation yet suffer untold complications—even fatal complications—if the nurses rendering postoperative care are not equally as competent and knowledgeable. By the same token, the most competent and knowledgeable nurses cannot prevent the problems that ensue from a surgeon who is not competent and knowledgeable.

Obviously the ideal setting is one in which nursing and medicine achieve a good balance, with practitioners within each exhibiting clinical expertise.

Obviously the ideal setting is one in which nursing and medicine achieve a good balance, with practitioners within each exhibiting clinical expertise. Such is not the case in most instances, however, and the imbalance gives rise to tensions, regardless of which shows more expertise. In situations where medicine excels and nursing does not, the nurse administrator can expect to experience enormous amounts of criticism and pressure for improvement from the medical staff. These criticisms are difficult to handle, indeed, and may even be the cause of a director's ultimate replacement should he or she fail to bring the department up to standard.

The converse situation may, however, prove to be equally if not more troublesome. If nursing excels and medicine does not, not only will the director receive vociferous demands from the nursing staff to press for improvements on the part of the physicians, but the latter will become threatened by the nurses and engage in efforts designed to curtail and diminish nursing practice.

In any case, the interdependence factor is one that is quite fluid, varying from time to time and from unit to unit. It requires from the nurse administrator an array of leadership behaviors that will assist in the restoration of the balance between the two professions and the preservation of nursing's autonomy.

SMALL GROUP BEHAVIOR

Another factor to be considered is the internal environment within the individual nursing unit. Because of the 24-hour nature of the work and because there must necessarily be a high degree of interdependence among various members of the nursing staff, interpersonal relations play an exceedingly important part in the delivery of care to patients. Thus the extent to which any individual can make a contribution is not solely dependent on clinical competence, but is also directly related to an ability to function well in small groups.

The problems of the small groups invariably become problems for the nurse administrator. Depending on the size of the institution and the administrator's own personal leadership style, she or he will become either directly or indirectly involved in attempting to build intraunit groups that function smoothly and harmoniously. Skill and ability in this area can do a great deal to further programmatic developments in clinical practice.

Nature of the External Environment: External Controls and Regulation

Undoubtedly the single most important feature in the external environment with which the nurse administrator must contend is that of external controls and regulation. While there has been considerable attention given to these in virtually every type of communication medium, their impact is becoming more severe and constraining every day. A study released in September of last year by the Hospital Association of New York State indicated that hospitals in New York State are inspected and/or regulated by 164 external agencies.[9]

Most recently, of course, the emphasis on cost containment has become the cause célèbre of the day. The fact that nursing represents the largest budget item for any inpatient facility makes that department the prime target for attack. Furthermore, because nursing is highly labor intensive, the attack is directed at personnel rather than at other expense items. The administrator is told by some regulatory agencies that a decrease in costs must ultimately mean a reduction in staff.

On the other hand, other regulatory agencies charged with responsibility for monitoring the quality of services rendered to patients frequently visit the same facilities and impose standards that essentially demand increases in staff in order for compliance to be achieved. Interestingly enough, it is not unusual for these contradictory and mixed messages to be coming from separate arms of the same parent organization (for example the federal or state government).

In such an environment, the nurse administrator must constantly be prepared to defend the function and organization of the department, using sound analytical approaches that employ both administrative and clinical knowledge.

Understanding some of the unique properties of the nurse administrator's role provides illumination of the areas to be considered in preparing individuals for a career in this field.

EDUCATIONAL PREPARATION FOR THE NURSE ADMINISTRATOR

For many years there has been a good deal of discussion and debate as to the type of preparation that is appropriate for the nurse administrator. In examining this problem, it becomes possible to envision the various points of view on a continuum as follows. (See Figure 1.) At the one

FIGURE. 1. CONTINUUM OF TYPE OF PREPARATION PROPOSED FOR NURSE ADMINISTRATORS

Master's In Business Admin.	Master's In Health Care Admin.	Master's In Nursing Combined With Health Care Admin.	Master's In Nursing Service Admin.	Master's In Nursing With Clinical Specialty

extreme are those who believe that the nurse administrator should have a master's degree in business administration; at the other extreme are those who believe the nurse administrator should have a master's degree in nursing, with clinical specialist preparation. Falling in between the two are those who believe in a master's degree in health care administration, a master's degree in nursing in combination with health care administration and a master's degree in nursing administration per se.

Those who are inclined toward favoring preparation in M.B.A. or M.H.A. programs make a case for the fact that the nurse is first and foremost an administrator and should be prepared as such. They believe that there is a need for in-depth study of the quantitative aspects of the position, with detailed course work in accounting and other budgeting aspects included. In fact, many hospital administrators and even some directors of nursing subscribe to this point of view. This may not be surprising if one understands that hospital administrators have their earliest roots in the business manager role[10] and that this continues to be of prime concern to them today. Directors of nursing, on the other hand, probably tend to overemphasize the need for such knowledge because they see this aspect as most troublesome to them, given the nature of the external environment at this point in time.

The problem with pursuing a purely administrative graduate preparation, however, should be obvious. It implicitly negates the fact that there might be content in *nursing* at the graduate level that the nurse administrator needs and should have. The message is clear: basic preparation in nursing is adequate for the nursing administrator; any additional knowledge in nursing that the administrator may need can be gained through continuing education.

In fact, quite the opposite is true. The director of nursing's primary responsibility is to give leadership to nursing through the use of administrative skills and knowledge. The director needs an intense, advanced-level study of nursing as well as course work in administration. Thus a combination of the two is an absolute requirement. As an aside, it should be

The director of nursing's primary responsibility is to give leadership to nursing through the use of administrative skills and knowledge.

noted that no medical center searches for a medical director whose only preparation beyond medical school is in administration.

In examining this issue, it becomes possible to draw an analogy between the preparation for the practice of nursing administration and the preparation for nursing in general. Most nurses and nonnurses alike would agree that nursing is more than an accumulation of the sciences that underlie its practice. In order to deal with the nursing needs of a 17-year-old quadriplegic, the nurse needs more than knowledge of the principles of physiology, pharmacology, physics, psychology and sociology; the whole is greater than the sum of its parts. So, too, is the practice of nursing administration more than a sum of personnel administration, budgeting, organizational behavior, etc. Because of its unique properties, the practice of nursing requires unique preparation; likewise, because of its unique properties, the practice of nursing administration requires unique preparation.

In addition, the paucity of research in the area of nursing administration speaks clearly to the need for doctoral preparation in this area. The fact that theories from other disciplines may be used in the field does not in any way indicate that these are sufficient to the task at hand. Many middle range theories need further explication before they can be meaningful to the practice field.[11] Most of this explication must be provided by nurse researchers who are also nurse administrators simply because others have neither the knowledge nor the interest to ask the pertinent, relevant questions. In this way a theoretical foundation can be laid for both the education and the practice of the nurse administrator.

Perhaps the best way to summarize the role of the director of nursing is to say that it is highly eclectic and highly complicated, and is becoming more so every day. The preparation of individuals to fill this role is therefore difficult at best. It would probably never be possible to develop a program that would encompass all the necessary knowledge and skills in a reasonable period of time. The challenge will be to set priorities for the content that are rational and practical.

REFERENCES

1. Thompson, J. D. *Organizations in Action* (New York: McGraw-Hill 1967).
2. Kinsella, C. R. *Nursing Service Administration: The State of the Art.* Paper prepared for Nursing and Health Care Administration Conference, Washington, D.C., January 1976, p. 4.
3. McClure, M. L. "The Long Road to Accountability." *Nursing Outlook* 26:1 (1978) p. 49.
4. Stromberg, M. F. "Relationship of Sex Role Identity to Occupational Image of Female Nursing Students." *Nursing Research* 25:5 (1976) p. 363–369.

5. Hennig, M. and Jardin, A. *The Managerial Woman* (Garden City, N.Y.: Anchor Press/Doubleday 1977).
6. Drucker, P. F. *Managing for Results* (New York: Harper & Row 1964).
7. Cleland, V. S. "Role Bargaining for Working Wives." *American Journal of Nursing* 70:6 (1970) p. 1242–1246.
8. Breslin, J. *How the Good Guys Finally Won: Notes from an Impeachment Summer* (New York: Ballantine Books 1975).
9. Hospital Association of New York State. *Report of the Task Force on Regulation* (Albany: HANYS 1978).
10. Arndt, C. and Huckabay, L. M. D. *Nursing Administration: Theory for Practice with a Systems Approach* (Saint Louis: The C. V. Mosby Co. 1975).
11. Thompson. *Organizations in Action.*

GROUP DISCUSSION

The Administrative Component

The following summarizes the group discussions on the administrative components of the nurse administrator's role, which took place at the Boston University School of Nursing conference.

Objectives

The objectives for the work session were:

1. to identify the major issues underlying the administrative component of the nurse administrator's role;
2. to develop a rationale for selecting each issue;
3. to identify the implications of each issue; and
4. to develop educational strategies and/or recommendations for the future.

Three critical issues were identified and the rationale for the selection and the implications of each were articulated. Educational strategies and recommendations were made in relation to the three issues.

Issue 1: Effective Utilization of Power

RATIONALE

Nursing administrators function within a political system and, in order to be effective, must understand and accept this as a fact and develop skill in using power strategically.

IMPLICATIONS

The risk exists that unless the issue of power is dealt with, nursing administration, or even nursing itself, may not survive as an identifiable, visible component of the health care system.

Utilization of power strategies is essential if nurse administrators are to have significant input into future solutions for health care excellence and delivery systems—both within their own agencies and at state and national levels.

Power, politics, authority and socialization are intertwined and all must be part of the nurse administrator's intellectual and action armamentarium.

There must be recognition of knowledge as one source of power.

There is an urgent need for nurse administrators who are educated, articulate professionals who speak and write for and about nursing.

Nurse administrators must develop the ability to be assertive and to use constructive confrontation and other adaptive behaviors.

The executive nurse administrator must be a member of the executive committee of the agency.

Nurse administrators must identify and use the locus of power as well as develop their own power base.

Alignment with power groups is imperative. These include boards of trustees and coalitions of nursing with consumers, with the medical profession, with subsystems and with other nursing groups.

Models of shared governance need to be developed.

A sound knowledge of management–labor relations is essential.

Issue 2: Effects of Budgetary and Quality Controls on the Professional Nursing Program

RATIONALE

The nurse administrator is responsible for supplying the human resources needed for provision of quality, cost-effective nursing care for patients and families. External agencies at all levels are promoting regulations relative to both cost containment and quality controls to which nurse administrators must be responsive. These regulations however, often seem to have conflicting impact on the nursing program.

IMPLICATIONS

Nurse administrators must have full control of the nursing budget, must be fiscally knowledgeable and articulate and able to develop, justify, defend and monitor the budget. It is also imperative that they be well informed about the fiscal aspects of the health care system at local, state and federal levels.

The relationship of program objectives to budget must be clearly defined and interpreted.

Nursing must be viewed as an income-generating service rather than just a cost factor. This requires competent, concentrated effort to define and measure nursing care and the establishment of financial rates for varying amounts and kinds of care.

The fact that few criterion measures of nursing care exist places emphasis on the need to replicate research studies and to develop additional criterion measures.

Patient classification systems need to be further refined and more widely utilized.

Staffing models which enhance both quality of care and productivity of nurses should be developed and tested.

Nurse administrators must have the authority to recruit qualified nursing personnel in accordance with the needs of the nursing program.

Recruitment, utilization, retention and development of staff are human resource factors influencing budget development and implementation.

Increased fiscal accountability should be required of staff. This requires a decentralized organization with delegation of budgetary responsibility to the unit level.

Nurse–consumer coalitions need to be created for the purpose of discussing and interpreting the expectations which both the public and the profession have regarding nursing care.

Issue 3: Nursing as a Subsystem of the Larger System of Health Care

RATIONALE

Nursing cannot survive in isolation. Its continuing existence and enrichment depend upon its interrelationships with other subsystems.

If nurse administrators are to survive the changing demands placed upon them by complex, multifarious issues, problems, programs, relationships and regulations within and without the agency, they must have knowledge and understanding of the overall health care system and nursing's place in it.

IMPLICATIONS

Nurse administrators must look beyond their own agencies to identify and interpret the role and contributions of nursing as a professional subsystem within the overall health care system.

The role of nursing must be interpreted to nurses themselves as well as to members of other subsystems.

Nurse administrators must be able to speak the language of other subsystems and multidisciplinary groups such as rate-setting commissions and health insurance agencies.

Decisions which may affect other subsystems are frequently made by the nurse administrator.

Particularly in large complex health care institutions, nurse administrators are bombarded with constantly changing demands which arise from multiple interfaces within the health care system. In order to cope with and adapt to these demands, a constant, sensitive changing of gears is required. A range of adaptive behaviors including assertiveness, confrontation and compromise must be part of the survival kit of the nurse administrator.

Knowledge and use of time management techniques may be helpful to survival in the demanding system.

Doctoral programs must be developed to prepare nurse administrators to function effectively within the complexities of the health care system.

Educational Strategies and Recommendations

Administration is an integral part of every professional role. It is imperative that increased recognition be given by the nursing profession in general and by all faculty members in particular, to nursing administration as a critical major area of study in nursing. Concepts must be introduced at the baccalaureate level and articulated with management/administration content at the master's and doctoral levels.

The educational goal for the top executive in nursing administration should be preparation at the doctoral level. However, the current paucity of those prepared at the master's or even at the baccalaureate level raises questions about the realism of that goal.

From the groups, the following recommendations emerged.

LEVELS OF PREPARATION

It is recommended that:

1. immediate emphasis be placed on the development of doctoral programs to prepare nurse executives for positions in large, highly complex health care facilities and to prepare researchers in nursing administration;
2. middle managers be prepared at the level of the master's program;
3. all clinical nurse specialist pro-

grams require a minor in nursing administration; and

4. the management process and its relationship to the nursing process be taught at the baccalaureate level.

EDUCATIONAL PROCESS

It is recommended that:

1. criteria for admission to nursing administration programs be refined to provide for the selection of appropriately qualified students;
2. there be a focus on the development of a knowledge base and administrative skills rather than on preparation for a specific role;
3. interface of nursing administration programs with other academic disciplines be expanded at both student and faculty levels;
4. teaching methodologies include case study and simulation training techniques; and
5. a clinical practicum introduce the student to the practice of nursing administration.

COLLABORATION BETWEEN NURSING EDUCATION AND NURSING SERVICE

It is recommended that:

1. nurse administrators provide input into the focus and content of educational programs;
2. nurse administrators develop a tangible sense of responsibility for the education of future nurse administrators;
3. nursing education and nursing service experiment with the development of different models for the student practicum;
4. preceptors be invited to attend university seminars;
5. faculty time be offered for staff education in preceptor's agency; and
6. experimental patient units be developed wherein faculty and students work with nursing service to help shape nursing care and nursing administration.

PROGRAM CONTENT

It is recommended that:

1. content in research methodology be included in the master's program and be a major focus of the doctoral program;
2. development of skill in small group work, including intergroup relationships, be given emphasis;
3. preparation for fiscal responsibility and accountability be given priority;
4. the theory and utilization of power be taught in the academic setting and followed up during the student's practicum;
5. the theory and application of the system's approach in health care delivery be taught;
6. the clinical practicum include the development of staffing patterns using the resources available, and following through with modifications, revisions and evaluation;
7. student experiences include involvement with various types of

nursing services, nursing service organizations and nursing systems as well as rate-setting bodies, boards of nursing meetings and other organizational activities; and

8. educational content of nursing administration programs which is needed for beginning functioning in nurse administrator role include: role theory; administrative-organizational theory; human behavior in organizations including small groups; research methodology; clinical components of the nurse administration role; political aspects of health care systems; development of quality assurance programs; human resources in health care organizations including recruitment, retention, utilization, evaluation, staff education, staffing and scheduling.

Clinical Nursing: A Basis for Administrative Excellence

Barbara Brown, R.N., Ed.D., F.A.A.N.
President
Hospital Administrative Assessment Profile, Inc.
Assistant Professor
Program in Nursing Administration
Community Health Care Systems
University of Washington
Seattle, Washington

NURSING—A CLINICAL SERVICE

NURSING, like medicine, is a clinical service, and it demands strong leadership by a qualified professional nurse who is prepared to integrate and apply knowledge of clinical nursing and management. The preparation of the nurse administrator must, therefore, blend an advanced level of clinical nursing knowledge and practice with the art and science of administration. This preparation will provide needed leadership in management of patient care, resources and finances.

Clinical practice frequently refers to the applications of theory and content of the fundamental sciences to the health care of clients. These sciences must be broadened in order to contrib-

This article is based on a presentation at "Nursing Administration: Directions for the Future," an invitational conference sponsored by the Boston University School of Nursing, November 3 and 4, 1978.

ute to the movement of clients and patients toward the desired health goals. Christman says that this process is "more than the mere gathering of scientific information and the glib use of it as professional rhetoric. It is a complex process that demands rigorous adherence to the methods of science in an orderly fashion."[1]

LEADERSHIP ROLE

Health care services will develop sound administrative planning *only* if the nurse administrator is able to bring effective leadership to the clinical practice of nursing and the patient care services rendered. An effective leader must have a broader knowledge base than do the persons being led.

Leadership in nursing administration means different things to nurses, physicians and administrators, depending on the tasks being performed at a given time. Nursing leadership is best described as the positive handling of professional interaction. The interactions between nursing and the medical staff, the administration and the patient require leadership which is based on knowledge, skill, experience, attitudes, responsibility, accountability and autonomy.

The nurse administrator must be creative and innovative. The courage of one's convictions, and the concern for all people may cause the administrator professional and personal risks. The nurse leader must be dedicated to the goals which the nurses are seeking and must demonstrate success in attaining these goals.[2]

GOALS OF NURSING

The goal of most professional nurses is to provide nursing care in an environment that enables them to fulfill their own potential as individual professionals. In order to create such an environment in professional practice, the nurse administrator must have a clinical nursing knowledge base.

The variations in education and experience that are found in clinical practice require the nurse administrator to have a deep understanding of clinical nursing. Administrators cannot continue to use graduates from all levels of basic nursing preparation equally—the professional and technical levels of clinical nursing practice should be differentiated more clearly. To understand and implement this differentiation, the curriculum in graduate education for nursing administration must include advanced nursing practice concepts.

Clinical nursing knowledge is needed to determine quality of patient care, standards for nursing practice, the role of the nurse, physician and nursing joint practice criteria and interdisciplinary health care standards.

COURSES IN CLINICAL NURSING

How much course work and practicum should constitute clinical nursing for nursing administration graduate students?

Students' chief area of preparation should be administration. Education, consultation, research and the service minor should also be included in their preparation. In planning their education, graduate students should be aware of their past education, experience and goals. Students whose clinical expertise and goals focus on care of children should have the opportunity to advance their clinical nursing knowledge base in that field. This would afford administrative leadership in pediatric settings.

Clinical theory and management practice sequences should be available in the maternal-child, psychiatric, geriatric and community health options. The practice component should combine clinical nursing knowledge with management knowledge and apply them to patient-care resources and fiscal affairs.

A systems approach could assist students to design clinical programs of services which are nursing oriented. The total management sequence of planning, organizing, staffing, budgeting, evaluating, researching, marketing and presenting a clinical nursing service to administration prepares the student for applying both clinical and administrative knowledge to a patient-care situation. This process would also involve planning and decision making by medical staffs, department heads from other disciplines and boards of trustees.

CLINICAL NURSING VALUES

The organizations in which most nurse administrators work are very complex. They demand high level management skills, respect of human beings and productivity, and a philosophy of nursing excellence. The attitudes, beliefs and values of clinical nursing practice must provide the focus for the future.

The philosophical base for nursing practice, which provides direction to the services rendered by nurses, requires that the nurse administrator be able to communicate the development and implementation of that nursing clinical practice.

It is well recognized that "in hospitals, nurses are the only professional workers providing a continuous and direct caring service. Care is a concept implying a measure of constancy and continuity." These two aspects, reinforced by communication, coordination, education and empathy, are the main components in nurses' contribution to care.[3]

In *Nursing Outlook*, January 1978, Jacox addressed the next generation of nurses, emphasizing that although nursing administrators are not generally members of top administration, they are largely responsible for the technical competence of nursing staff. The increasing proliferation of hospital administrators has resulted in many of the functions formerly performed by nursing administrators now being carried out by others. These include personnel management, budgeting, negotiating with labor unions, evaluating nurses' efficiency, and handling malpractice problems.[4]

HOSPITAL ADMINISTRATION

The proliferation of hospital administrators (which may include former

The proliferation of hospital administrators will lead to the removal of nurse leaders from top nursing executive positions—if nurses allow that to happen.

occupational therapists, pharmacists, insurance personnel, personnel managers and former nurses) *will* lead to the removal of nurse leaders from top nursing executive positions in health care delivery systems—if nurses allow that to happen.

In the autumn of 1978, the American Hospital Association (AHA) took a significant action regarding the executive role of the nurse administrator. The AHA endorsed the *Statement on Role, Functions, and Qualifications of the Nursing Service Administrator in a Health Care Institution.*

This statement, developed by the AHA Committee on Nursing and the American Society for Nursing Service Administrators, calls for a synthesis of clinical background and management skills in preparing the nursing service administrator to be an effective manager of the department of nursing and to represent staff and patients at the same time.[5]

The AHA described nursing administrative responsibilities as follows:

- developing policies and procedures that govern the nursing service in collaboration with appropriate services;
- defining and maintaining the standards of nursing practice within the institution; and
- assessing the quality of care rendered by the nursing service.

The AHA continued:

> The principal colleagues of nursing service administrators are chief executive officers, chief medical officers, and the other members of the management team of the institution. Nursing service administrators have the responsibility of interpreting and representing nursing to all other departments of the health care institution. Nursing service administrators should appropriately participate at the Board level and with the medical staff in the formulation of policies that affect the nursing service.
>
> Nursing service administrators have a responsibility to represent nursing in the local community and to promote continuity of care between the institutions and other health care providers in the community. They also share nursing's traditional advocacy of patients' rights. As leaders in the profession, they establish, monitor, and support standards of nursing practice. They also provide for the initiation, support, and/or evaluation of needed research.
>
> Nursing service administrators need a strong personal and professional commitment to the practice of nursing service administration. They accept the responsibility to practice their profession according to the highest ethical standards. They must hold a current license from the state in which they practice.[6]

IMPLICATIONS FOR THE FUTURE

What are the implications for the future preparation of nursing administration?

First, the administrator of nursing services must be a registered professional nurse. Administration of nursing services requires advanced clinical nursing knowledge and cannot be relegated to proliferating hospital administrators.

Also, managing personnel, evaluating nurses' efficiency, budgeting and staffing must be the major work of the nurse administrator.

Therefore, our task is to prepare nurses to become administrators who, through a synthesis of clinical nursing and management knowledge and practice, can combine the role of professional nurse and professional manager.

"Nurses must assume a more visible and vital leadership role in the delivery of health care if nursing is to remain a viable profession."[7] This visible and vital role takes place within the organizational setting, the community at large and the political arena. Nurse administrators can provide significant input in decision making for health care priorities. Clinically sophisticated nurse managers will develop programs of services for hospitalized patients as well as community-based services and will be the primary force in reshaping health care delivery systems. "Nursing needs to and is going to take over the health care system."[8]

POTENTIAL FOR CHANGE

With expert clinical knowledge as the base of power, nursing has the potential to organize massive change. A nurse administrator who is clinically sophisticated in knowledge and practice components and who uses a creative approach can increase services which focus on the uniqueness of nursing practice. These services, which are being demanded by consumers, are based on patient education and health promotion.

With expert clinical knowledge as the base of power, nursing has the potential to organize massive change.

Nursing can take over the health care system on behalf of the consumer through implementation of clinical nursing services such as sexual assault treatment centers; cardiopulmonary rehabilitation and prevention programs; comprehensive diabetic, arthritic, pain and geriatric centers; child-abuse programs; and family-centered nursing programs in pediatrics, maternity, general medical–surgical and psychiatry.

"The proper focus for the development of nursing knowledge is nursing practice."[9] A nursing administrator must create an environment which encourages the full practice of professional nursing. Without an advanced clinical nursing knowledge base, this would be most difficult.

PROFESSIONAL NURSE ROLES

How many present nursing administrators expect the full implementation of professional nursing practice from the nurses they employ? Nurse administrators and staff must believe that the nurse's basic principle of being is to give direct *service* to patients, i.e., direct patient care. We cannot afford to prostitute the role

FIGURE 1. THE ROLE OF THE RN

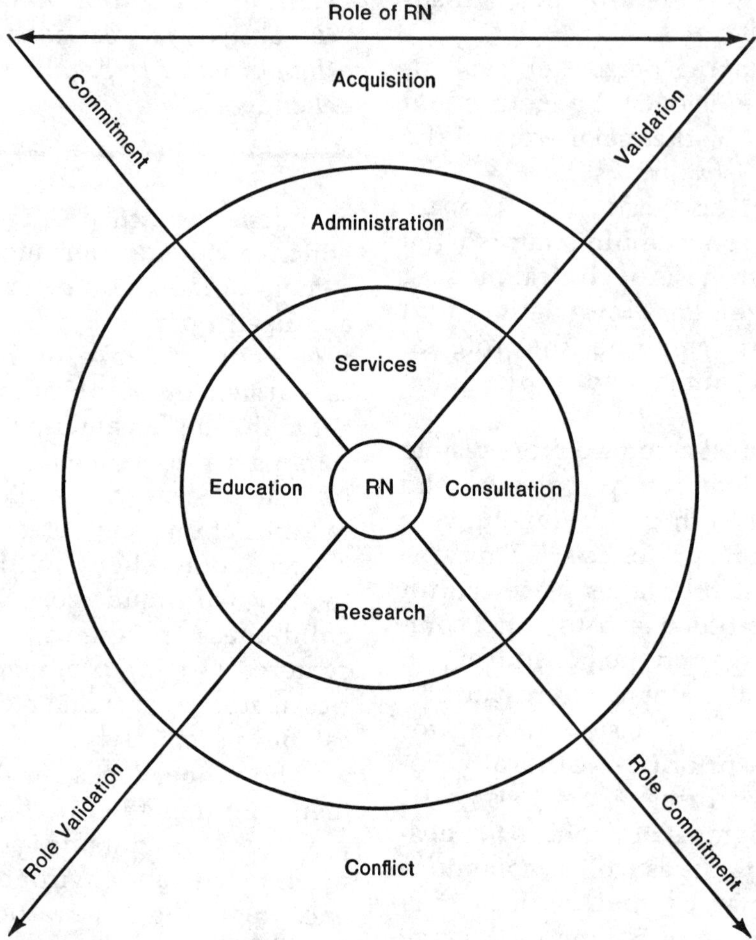

Role acquisition occurs in two basic ways: role validation and role commitment. Role validation is behavior which meets community expectation. Role commitment is adoption of behavior that best represents the role model the person wishes to occupy. Conflict occurs when the community entertains expectations which the individual feels unable to realize.

relationship between the patient and the nurse by putting layers of others between the patient and the nurse. Nurses must *teach* patients as much about their health status as possible. This teaching role of nurses takes place when nurses are direct care givers.

Nurses are also *consultants*. In this capacity they share expertise with colleagues on a one-to-one basis and refer to clinical experts to meet the nursing needs of patients. Physicians refer patients to other physicians when there is a medical need for consultation. Nurses should refer patients to other nurses when necessary.

The *research* role is necessary in order to change the direction of nursing practice. Every nurse should be applying research findings to practice to enhance the wellness of each individual patient and family constellation.[10]

Nursing administrators perform the administrative role as a major nursing component in order to facilitate the achievement of the other four roles of professional nursing. (See Figure 1.)

The nurse administrator focuses on the administrative role in order to create a quality patient care system. This patient care system depends on comprehensive clinical nursing knowledge and practice.

The ANA Commission on Nursing Services, in *Roles, Responsibilities and Qualifications for Nurse Administrators,* states that the background of nurse administrators must include "such clinical and administrative practice as to lead to the consistent fulfillment of each responsibility inherent in the respective administrative role."[11]

POWER BASE

"The critical challenge facing nursing over the next 25 years will be to acquire a solid resource and power base upon which to move the profession forward."[12] The power base that is needed for nursing has to do with both position and knowledge. More than 7,000 nurses have the position power base as directors of nursing services. The development of these services is dependent upon a high level of nursing knowledge and practice.

With the knowledge power base of clinical nursing gained through graduate education, nursing can give direction to the future health care delivery systems. How the clinical nursing power base is built through the development of excellence in nursing service administration will shape the future of nursing.

"We shape our buildings; thereafter they shape us."[13]

—Winston Churchill

REFERENCES

1. Christman, L. "Accountability and Autonomy Are More Than Rhetoric." *Nurse Education* (July-August 1978) p. 4.
2. Brown, B. J. "Leadership in Nursing Administration." *Nursing Administration Quarterly* 1:1 (Fall 1976) p. v.
3. Hockey, L. "The Nurse's Contribution to Care in a Changing Setting." *Journal of Advanced Nursing* 2: (March 1977) p. 147–156.
4. Jacox, A. "Address to the Next Generation." *Nursing Outlook* (January 1978) p. 39.
5. American Hospital Association. "Statement on Role, Functions, and Qualifications of the Nursing Service Administrator in a Health Care Institution" approved by House of Delegates, 1978.
6. Ibid.
7. Jacobi, E. M. "The Moral Leadership of the Nursing Profession." *Journal of Advanced Nursing,* 2: (November 1977) p. 561–569.
8. Diers, D. "A Different Kind of Energy: Nurse-Power" *Nursing Outlook* (January 1978) p. 52.
9. Ibid. p. 54.
10. Brown, B. J. "Affecting Nursing Goals in Health Care." *Nursing Administration Quarterly* 2:3 (Spring 1978) p. 27–28.
11. American Nurses' Association, Commission on Nursing Services. *Roles, Responsibilities, and Qualifications for Nurse Administrators* (1978) p. 14.
12. Kalisch, B. J. "The Promise of Power." *Nursing Outlook* (January 1978) p. 43.
13. Peter, L. J. The Peter Prescription (New York: Bantam Books 1972) p. 214.

GROUP DISCUSSION

Clinical Components

The following summarizes the group discussions on the clinical components of the nursing administrator's role, which took place at the Boston University School of Nursing conference.

Objectives

The objectives for the work session were:

1. to identify the major issues underlying the clinical component of the nurse administrator's role;
2. to develop a rationale for each issue;
3. to identify the implications of each issue; and
4. to develop educational strategies and/or recommendations for the future.

Three major issues were identified. In discussing the first two issues, the rationale and implications were considered together and both positive and negative aspects were articulated. Educational strategies and recommendations apply to the three issues.

Issue 1: Appropriateness of the Clinical Component in Nursing Administration Programs

Traditionally, the clinical component has not been part of graduate programs in nursing administration. However, the clinical component is now appropriate for the following reasons. [Note: there was marked lack of consensus among group members particularly regarding whether or not graduate students in nursing administration programs need direct experience in advanced clinical nursing practice.]

1. Nurse administrators need to have a clinical knowledge base because they manage the clinical practice of others.
2. The discipline of nursing administration is nursing, and programs preparing nurse administrators must advance the knowledge base of nursing.
3. A clinical knowledge base increases one's ability to communicate with nursing as a profession as well as with other health-related disciplines.
4. The majority of hospitals in the United States have less than 100 beds and, in these smaller institutions, the nurse administrator may be the only qualified, clinical resource person.
5. To create an environment for nursing practice in which professionals have accountability and credibility, the nurse administrator needs a general understanding of advanced clinical practice.

The clinical component may be inappropriate for the following reasons.

1. A learner may have had extensive clinical practice and may already be a competent practitioner.
2. Some positions, such as those in Health Maintenance Organizations (HMOs), may not require specific clinical knowledge.

3. Economy of time, energy and finances presents realistic constraints in program design. The inclusion of a clinical component may compromise the priority for a deeper knowledge of nursing administration content.
4. If a clinical component is included, means by which the nurse administrator would maintain current clinical knowledge, and still have time to maintain and advance knowledge in administration, must be found.

Issue 2: Purpose of the Clinical Component

The purpose of the clinical component is to assist nurse administrators to:

1. assimilate concepts of advanced nursing knowledge and/or advanced clinical nursing practice;
2. increase credibility in their position;
3. appreciate the depth of knowledge and skill of the nursing staff under their direction as well as improve their perceptions of nursing administration;
4. become involved with education and clinical research programs;
5. interpret nursing to nurses, consumers and other health disciplines; and
6. provide leadership in quality assurance programs.

There was consensus that the purpose of the clinical component is *not* to prepare nurse administrators who are also clinical specialists.

Issue 3: Nature of the Clinical Component

Discussion focused largely on attempts to define the clinical component. No consensus was reached concerning a definition, but the following three dimensions of the component were debated: provision of direct nursing care enabling the student to apply clinical knowledge and theory to practice; knowledge of advanced clinical concepts related to synthesis in practice; and advanced clinical knowledge relating to clinical issues.

It was agreed that the assessment of the clinical background which each individual student brings to the educational program will help determine the nature of the clinical component for that student.

Two sets of implications, representing diverse opinions with regard to the nature and focus of the clinical component, were outlined: specific focus and broad, general focus.

Positive implications of *specific focus* include:

- Viewing and studying a specific patient population serves as a vehicle for accruing content and process which can be transferred to other populations.
- Specific focus provides for economy of time in the educational program.
- Specific focus provides options to career possibilities.

A *negative* implication of this approach may be that the student develops too narrow a perspective of clinical knowledge and application.

Positive implications of *broad, general focus* on key, clinical concepts include:

- It develops the ability to blend a clinical and an administrative role.
- It provides career options which may be desirable at a later date.
- It provides for economy of time, energy and money by focusing on key concepts applicable to all clinical areas.
- It promotes the use of many key clinical concepts in administrative practice.
- It prepares the learner to identify key points in resolving issues in the administration of complex situations.

Negative implications include:

- Emphasis may be so broad that assimilation of essential principles and concepts is difficult.
- Learners may be unable to identify clinical knowledge which is relevant to administration.

Educational Strategies and Recommendations

It is recommended that:

1. the clinical component provide an understanding of the method of studying clinical phenomena;
2. terminal, behavioral objectives for the clinical component be defined in collaboration with clinical experts;
3. based on the students' background and goals, options be available for the attainment of advanced clinical knowledge.
4. the development of clinical proficiency examinations be given consideration.
5. key clinical concepts be identified in collaboration with clinical experts.
6. the nurse administrator develop an understanding of clinical phenomena and language.

There was lack of consensus among group members as to the means by which this ability should be achieved. Some members believed that the ability to conceptualize clinical phenomena is the essential indication of the nurse administrator's knowledge of clinical content. Other members are convinced that without direct patient care contact in a clinical practicum, the nurse administrator can neither use clinical language nor conceptualize clinical phenomena.

Knowledge Generation and Transmission: A Role for the Nurse Administrator

Mary E. Conway, Ph.D., R.N., F.A.A.N.
Dean, School of Nursing
Medical College of Georgia
Augusta, Georgia
Former Dean, School of Nursing
University of Wisconsin-Milwaukee
Milwaukee, Wisconsin

THE TITLE of this article is suggestive. It suggests that there is a role for the nurse administrator in both the generation of knowledge and its transmission. Yet there are a number of assumptions implicit in this declaration which have not been made explicit, nor have nurse administrators attempted to discover among themselves as professionals to what extent they support them. Rather than explore these assumptions, however, it is more fruitful to begin a consideration of the role of nurse administrators with respect to both of these functions by asking the broader question, What expectations *should* nurse administrators have for themselves as a body of expert professionals? And what do the

This article is based on a presentation at "Nursing Administration: Directions for the Future," an invitational conference sponsored by the Boston University School of Nursing, November 3 and 4, 1978.

consumers or potential consumers of their expert services *demand* of them?

Knowledge is the unique characteristic of the 20th century. The pace of knowledge generation is the most salient feature of the latter part of this century, and the unique ability of our society to use knowledge clearly has resulted in technological advances unthought of 30 years ago—or only hinted at in science fiction—and a bettering of the human condition exceeding the previous generation's most utopian imagination. Yet these impressive achievements are accompanied by such undesirable side effects as an increasing death rate from accidents, an increasing incidence of drug and alcohol dependence, a high proportion of obesity among the adult population, an increase in suicide among adolescents and a stubbornly high unemployment rate among minority groups—particularly the black population. The fact is that the benefits of a high-technology society accrue unevenly both to those who help make the technology possible and those who are the consumers of its output. Nowhere is this uneven impact more apparent than in the health care field where the lower income segment of the population still has reduced access to care, as well as inferior or incomplete care in those places it is accessible. These undesirable features of our social world suggest that (1) our knowledge is still so incomplete as to preclude altering these patterns, (2) we have not as yet applied existing knowledge to alter them and/or (3) we are unwilling to alter them. Any one of these possibilities is of concern. From the few examples cited above it is evident that in spite of its potential for high pay-off, knowledge is not uniformly utilized to solve all the social problems it is potentially capable of solving, nor is it utilized by as many policy makers as there are who have access to it.

Administrators of social institutions are a special class of knowledge utilizers; nurse administrators, a subclass of all administrators, then by extension are also knowledge utilizers. In fact, it is reasonable to say that they represent a unique class of administrators. They are legitimate in administrative roles for one important reason: they possess a body of knowledge unique to a science-based discipline—*nursing*. Their abilities as administrators serve—or should serve—to safeguard and extend the specialized knowledge that is nursing to those clients who are in need of it.

If we were to examine a hierarchical order of role expectations for nurse administrators it would become apparent that the demands for those role behaviors attached to the broad administrative functions of the organization take precedence over those attached to "protection" and "extension" of the professional service component. At the top of a theoretical hierarchy of demands placed upon administrators in general is the requirement that stability of the organization be maintained.[1,2] This requirement may bear little relationship to the hands-on activities that comprise the specialized professional service given to the clients who are the organization's raison d'etre. Katz and Kahn assert that mechanisms that maintain stability attempt to institutionalize the organization's behaviors. Standardizing operations thereby reduces behavioral choices and enhances stability.[3]

The position that all human behavior within organizations tends to be prescribed, ritualized and formalized irrespective of the organization's specific purpose for existing is supported by a number of other researchers.[4-6] This reality has important implications for nursing and nurse administrators. It suggests, for example, that nurse administrators will have to exert additional effort over and above the normative expectations of their roles *as administrators* to ensure that their specialized discipline (nursing) is represented to clients in its optimal form and provided by competent practitioners.

However, a large number of nurse administrators are not capable of carrying out this latter role function. There are two principal reasons for this: (1) many nurses occupying administrator roles have had insufficient formal preparation for the administrator role and (2) many have not had professional-level preparation in nursing, or have had incomplete preparation. The combined effects of one or both of these variables are evident in the numbers of nurses who are ineffective administrators, allowing their sphere of professional work autonomy to be invaded or controlled by nonqualified administrators. To some extent this unjustified incursion by others into what is appropriately a nursing decision-making sphere is invited by nurse administrators who are unable to communicate clearly the justification and rationale for their own decision making. Again, knowledge is the keystone of an evolved society, and nurse administrators (among others) have an obligation to safeguard and provide for the transmission of that unique body of knowledge which is nursing.

THE QUESTION

To what extent can knowledge generation be considered a legitimate part of role expectations for nurse administrators? And, given that there is a role, what is its nature?

To what extent can knowledge generation be considered a legitimate part of role expectations for nurse administrators? And, given that role, what is its nature?

NURSING AS SCIENCE

Science is knowledge. Knowledge consists of certain coded facts within the head from which connections are made to certain realities existing outside of the head—that is, to phenomena which are the features of existence.[7] The more closely the patterns in the mind parallel the real world, the "more empirically useful and valid the science."[8] Nursing is science in that researchers and practitioners of the discipline constantly endeavor to organize the phenomena of human behavior in meaningful patterns, devise interventions on the basis of these organizing attempts and evaluate the outcomes. While much of the organizing and interventions are devised on the basis of thoughtful analysis, much of the effort to know that which is unknown takes place as research.

Ten years ago Schrag observed that the behavioral disciplines and the helping professions in general made limited use of research strategies.[9] That statement does not apply to the behavioral sciences today. Behavioral sciences are among the leading professional disciplines contributing to the development of useful knowledge through research.

Nursing, as a science, is at the frontier of its discoveries. Some would challenge this assertion claiming that nursing's science is well established.[10,11] There are two principal reasons that nursing is at the frontier of its discoveries; one is that research by nurses *in* nursing is just now reaching sizable proportions; the other is that there still exists a wide gap between the domains of research and practice.

Obviously, since the ultimate test of knowledge is its application, this gap poses problems for the evolution of nursing's practice base. The findings which are generated by research provide the base for reconceptualizing nursing practice. Reconceptualization does not imply that practice requires a wholesale reconceptualization, but simply that practice must constantly be adjusted to take into account newer knowledge and more effective interventions based on such knowledge.

For example, one alteration in practice which is likely to occur over time as more knowledge is gained is in the direction of applying more generalized interventions to aggregates as opposed to the prevailing focus on individualized interventions. Also, we will have more knowledge about which input variables are directly correlated with specific outcomes. An important task for nursing—perhaps its most important task as a learned discipline—is a continuing, rigorous reassessment of current knowledge upon which nursing practice is based. Schrag, in explicating the relationship between science and the helping professions noted that, for the practitioner, science is an enterprise and the vehicle through which inadequate current knowledge can be updated.[12]

It might be instructive to consider how closely nursing as a discipline approximates the ideal set of criteria by which a science is defined. There are five criteria by which science/nonscience can be defined: (1) a body of researchers exists; (2) the methods of the discipline involve the statement of theories; (3) these theories are tested and from them facts are deduced; (4) testing of the theories leads to the development of additional theories which in turn are subjected to test; and (5) findings are never considered incontrovertible but only hypothetical, as yet unfalsified. Theories, then, are the essence of any science and the practice of the discipline stems from them.

An important consideration for a practice discipline such as nursing is the fact that very often research does not deal with real-time and real-world conditions. Thus the extension of thought into action—that is, practice—may be delayed. Argyris and Schon consider the concept of rigorous research an obstacle to thought and action. They believe that self-fulfilling prophecies may have to be accepted because so-called rigorous research cannot cope with real time and environmental conditions.[13]

The second and third criteria enumerated above—the testing of theories and the methods of the discipline—deal with the *test of evidence.* That is, a theory will survive only to the extent that it is able to generate evidence in the real world which supports it. If for *no other* reason, the nurse researchers must insist on gaining access to the real-world laboratory since this is also the realm in which their research findings will be applied in practice.

AUTHORITY AS A REQUIREMENT FOR PROFESSIONAL PRACTICE

Nursing exhibits to a greater or lesser degree those criteria by which a science-based discipline is identified. There is an additional criterion by which the learned professions are identified and assigned value by consumers: *authority.* No discipline can hope to measure up to its full potential unless it possesses authority. By definition authority is that command of a body of knowledge and/or field of practice which is acknowledged as reserved to it by other professionals and consumers. Authority is manifest in a profession's control both of its practice and the standards it sets for entry into practice. Nursing's possession of authority is tenuous at best, and at worst, it is nonexistent in many practice settings.

Authority is that command of a body of knowledge and/or field of practice which is acknowledged as reserved to it by other professionals and consumers. It is manifest in a profession's control both of its practice and the standards it sets for entry into practice.

There are a number of reasons why this situation exists at the present time, some of which are commonly known. The most fundamental reason for nursing's lack of authority is that except for its earliest years it has been under the control of another profession. And while this dominance can be overcome with time as nursing continues to demonstrate its contribution to the public's health, in an ever-increasing number of arenas the process of emancipation will require a protracted effort.

Recent action taken by the profession's organizational voice to mandate a statutory level for entry into professional practice is an encouraging sign that nursing is moving ahead to control its practice. An additional movement which should be completed within the next five to six years—one intended to protect both the consumer and the practitioner—is the establishment of two licensing examinations: one to assess basic competency for technical level practice and one to assess competency for professional practice.

Nursing's lack of authority has at least contributed to, if not caused, a very real and serious problem for the credibility of the profession. This problem is manifest in those settings where the practice of nursing is the most visible to clients. The practice most visible to clients is that which takes place in hospitals and is the form which often bears the least resemblance to the profession's ideal prescriptions. (Ideal prescriptions are those statements made about the nature of a profession's practice which are promulgated to inform both the profession's practitioners and consumers of its service.) To be more explicit, the statements made by the official representatives of the profession about nursing practice do not coincide with the reality of the care provided to recipients. Thus there exists a serious credibility gap for the profession. This gap will not be reduced by continued statements unless those statements are accompanied by a visible alteration in the nature of the practice itself.

A regrettable consequence of this credibility gap is nursing's failure to obtain an optimal level of federal support for higher education in nursing. Some would argue that the failure to gain the necessary support may be related to the fact that some professionals—notably physicians—do recognize nursing's authority and are threatened by what they perceive as a lessening of their own sphere of authority if nurses are allowed to practice at the level their preparation warrants. To some extent both perceptions may coexist.

If both knowledge generation and real-world application are necessary conditions for a practice discipline's acquiring authority for its practice, what steps can nursing take to secure its authority? One step might be to construct a conceptual model which identifies the essential elements required for a science-based discipline intent on closing the loop from its Statement of Theories to Adoption-in-Practice of Its Prescriptions. Study of the model would suggest at what points specific outcomes are indicated. Such a model is presented in Figure 1.

The elements of the model are divided into three main categories: Prerequisite Conditions, Method and Application. The variables included in the category Prerequisite Conditions are the existence of a body of researchers and a body of practitioners and the statement of theories and development of conceptual frameworks. The category Method includes the formulation of hypotheses, the testing of hypotheses, the development of evidence, the making of prescriptive statements and further testing of

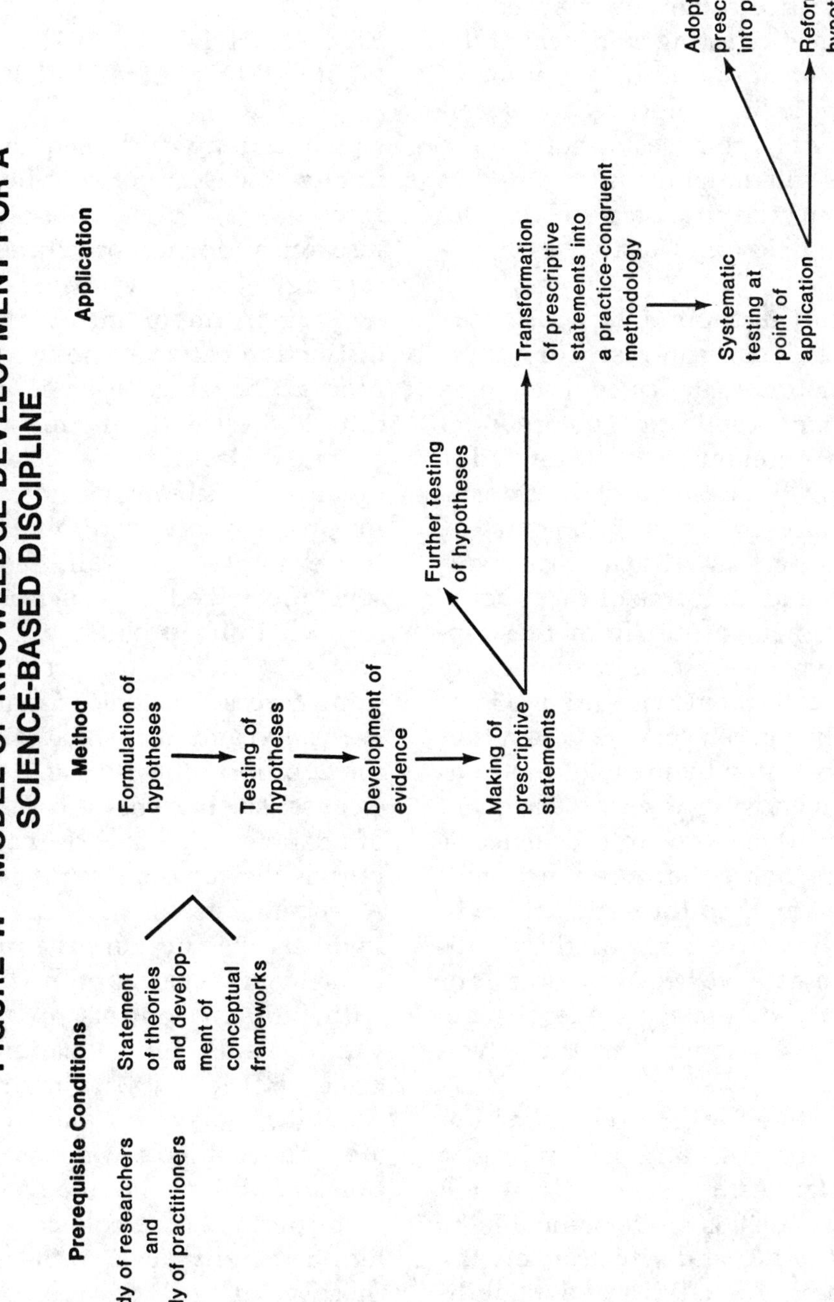

FIGURE 1. MODEL OF KNOWLEDGE DEVELOPMENT FOR A SCIENCE-BASED DISCIPLINE

hypotheses. In the category Application the following are included: transformation of prescriptive statements into a practice-congruent methodology, systematic testing and evaluation at point of application, adoption of prescriptions into practice and reformulation of hypotheses. Results of the latter are subsequently transmitted as feedback to the first step in Method: the formulation and testing of hypotheses.

That part of the model which may hold the most interest for nurse administrators is the category labeled Application. Application incorporates the vital elements of knowledge generation, education and the translation of prescriptions into practice. Knowledge is both a forerunner and an outcome of those activities that seek to transform prescriptive statements into a methodology which is congruent with the mode of practice in a given setting. One rather obvious reason why many of the findings from nursing research have not yet found their way into practice is that there has either been no well-developed method for testing them in real-practice situations, or the methods proposed have been too esoteric or alien to the customary mode of practice by practitioners in the given setting.

A challenge for both the researcher and the practitioner is finding a method for testing selected research findings which is understandable to the practitioner and which meets the requirements for validity and reliability. This effort when jointly undertaken by researchers and practitioners is knowledge generating in and of itself.

RESEARCH DIFFERENTIATED FROM PROBLEM SOLVING

A question which frequently arises in any discussion of so-called applied research is, What constitutes true research and what constitutes problem solving? There are several reasons why it is important to clarify the distinction between the two. First, the process by which each is conducted differs. Research (if the activity is properly classified as such) must be organized with a rigor not demanded for problem solving. Problem solving, for example, generally consists of some prescribed steps such as identifying what the problem is, gathering data surrounding the problem, examining forces that tend to maintain the status quo and forces that tend to alter the equilibrium; working at achieving a consensus on what the desired state of affairs *should* be; and finally taking purposive steps to alter the situation. A second reason is that research involves specification of a problem in terms such that an appropriate method with built in controls for reliability, validity and generalization can be constructed. Value positions—"shoulds"—have no place here. Data are collected according to specifications of the methodology employed and often must be collected by disinterested individuals rather than by those who will be affected by the outcomes. Thus it should be clear that method, validity and reliability are key elements of research but not necessarily of problem solving. The costs associated with each are likely to be very different; research in general is much more costly than problem solving.

In practical terms, a first step for nurse administrators and concerned nursing staffs who wish to bring about useful innovation or gain more knowledge about patient-related phenomena is to decide whether or not the phenomena to be studied fall within the classification of research or problem solving.

A first step for nurse administrators and concerned nursing staffs who wish to bring about useful innovation or gain more knowledge about patient-related phenomena is to decide whether or not the phenomena fall within the classification of research or problem solving.

There are several criteria which if applied to a question to be studied will yield the answer. Seven such criteria to distinguish research are: (1) the question cannot be answered by fact finding alone; (2) the problem and its "solution" are likely to yield important information applicable to a broad range of settings or populations; (3) any change in current practice recommended as a result of the investigation is applicable to all other classes of organizations or populations having like characteristics; (4) the "solution" is not apparent prior to the proposed investigation; (5) the problem is derived from or contributes to a theoretical framework; (6) validity and reliability can be assessed; and (7) the investigation is capable of replication by others.

MOVING TOWARD INSTITUTIONALIZATION OF RESEARCH IN PRACTICE SETTINGS

The identification of some pragmatic considerations involved in the institutionalization of research in practice settings in general can provide a focus or a catalyst for interesting discussion.

It should be acknowledged that two opposing cultures are being dealt with—a knowledge-generating culture and a knowledge-utilizing culture. The former is interested in truth, validity and discovery; the latter, in a process-oriented rationality and the feasible over the desirable.[14] There are bound to be strains between these two cultures, yet each has something to offer the other. It is in this overlapping area that nurse administrators will find it most useful to seek a compelling rationale for initiating and institutionalizing research. For example, what kinds of outcomes may be expected from research that are likely to be viewed as "goods" from both the knowledge-generating culture's perspective and the knowledge-utilizing culture's perspective? What is the appropriate starting point? How much should be attempted; that is, what should be the scope of the research endeavor? Who should be involved? What is timely? What resources are or can be made available? These are but a few of the questions that administrators will need to ask themselves.

Three variables are relevant to our question: state of the art, the nature of interprofessional relationships and the organization's orientation to its environment. Singly, and together, these variables are important "conditioners" of the environment in which research is ongoing or is anticipated.

STATE OF THE ART

In any specialized field of knowledge the type of research which is done is a reflection of the state of knowledge in that field. For example, prior to the development of the electron microscope the research which resulted in the identification of the genetic code (DNA) was not possible. Similarly, in nursing, until it is known which interventions are highly correlated with specific outcome criteria, experimental studies in which intervention is a variable cannot be conducted. There are a few notable exceptions, of course. Johnson, in her research on varying nursing interventions with patients undergoing threatening procedures, has demonstrated that individual response to threat can be reduced. Her study reveals that intervention which gives patients prior knowledge of sensations they will experience is associated with significant reduction in stress.[15]

Some areas which are being researched by nurses have evolved faster than others. One in which there has been considerable progress is that of evaluation research. The prominent example which comes to mind, of course, is quality assurance. In quality assurance studies, there is a great deal of data available on which outcome criteria are met more or less in a given setting. However, little or no correlation has been established between *process* and outcomes.[16,17] Another unknown is to what extent these outcomes correlate with the health status of clients after their discharge from the care setting. Scott, for example, notes that in evaluating the success of surgery it is insufficient to assess morbidity only seven days post surgery or at the time of discharge. There must be an assessment at a later point in time before any conclusion can be drawn about morbidity.[18] Still using the example of evaluation research, evaluation of nursing care relies upon process measures which in turn are derived from accepted standards, but we do not know how "correct" the standards themselves are.

Communication is a limiting factor at present in nursing research. A great deal of research is being done in a number of settings which as yet has not been disseminated, or its dissemi-

A great deal of research is being done in a number of settings which as yet has not been disseminated, or its dissemination is restricted to a limited geographic area.

nation is restricted to a limited geographic area. This situation, however, is being slowly remedied. Several new journals devoted to reporting research in nursing have been established over the past year and a half; this additional outlet should make research findings more readily accessible to the professional community.

In sum, what is possible in *type* of research to be undertaken and its *level* of sophistication depends upon the knowledge base provided by previous research.

NATURE OF INTERPROFESSIONAL RELATIONSHIPS

The second variable identified above is the nature of interprofessional relationships within the delivery setting. There is an infinite variation in these relationships; some of this variation is attributed to the size and complexity of the organization, the guiding ethos of the organization, the competence of the professionals who work in the organization and the degree of work autonomy allowed professionals. If we restrict ourselves to the relationships between nurses and physicians, it is apparent that research is more likely to flourish in those settings where a collegial relationship exists between each group, and where the efforts of each are overtly directed to serving the welfare of the client or patient. The reward structure of the organization in turn reinforces this latter dimension. If rewards are given for performance related to client welfare, such performance will be enhanced. Collegiality and client focus are circular in that one reinforces the other.

Organizations in which collegial relationships exist tend to be among the more prestigious and widely known to others outside the immediate environment. Hence they tend to draw competent professionals who wish to be associated with centers of excellence.[19]

If physicians tend to dominate a setting in such a way as to control or restrain the behavior of nurses, there can be no collegiality. In such settings, dependence on the part of nurses is fostered and critical peer review of professional performance will be negligible or nonexistent. Nursing practice in such settings, as is well known to informed observers, will reflect more of a medical orientation than patient-centered nursing practice.

Access to patients is controlled by physicians in hospital settings. This access must be extended to nurses if research is to take place. Since the process of gaining access will be facilitated in those settings where collegiality is already a norm, it will be in the interest of nurse administrators to enhance collegiality between nurses and physicians as a prior step to seeking access to patients for research. The administrator may have to serve as the exemplary role model in this effort.

THE ORGANIZATION'S ORIENTATION TO ITS ENVIRONMENT

Organizations differ in their relationship to their environments. Those which have more difficulty than others in obtaining scarce resources (money and qualified workers) will take fewer risks and tend to be more closed as a system. That is, they will not attempt innovation until and unless such innovation has been demonstrated elsewhere to be desirable. Organizations which gain reputations as leaders in innovation achieve this reputation on the basis of earlier risk taking and subsequent positive or approving feedback from their external environments. These conditions are usually present in hospitals and community-based health organizations.

Research, of course, would be viewed as an innovation by those organizations that are more closed than open systems. The task, therefore, for those who seek to introduce research is first to alter inputs into the organization in such a way as to alter throughput and ultimately output.

One possible way to alter the internal environment to make it more receptive to innovation (research) would be to seek a new or intensified collaboration with an organization in the external environment. Such collaboration will ultimately alter both input and throughput in the focal setting. For example, some health care settings, both hospital and community based, seek alliances with their nurse colleagues in a university. There are a number of places where this collaborative relationship continues strong and productive for both parties to the arrangement. Among successful models are Ohio State University, the University of Washington, the University of Arizona, the University of Michigan, Wayne State University and the University of Wisconsin at Milwaukee.

One strategy for attempting to "open" a setting to innovation might be to select a successful research study which has "paid off" in another

One strategy for attempting to "open" a setting to innovation might be to select a successful research study which has "paid off" in another setting and replicate it.

setting and replicate it. Assuming it pays off again on replication, this demonstration might provide sufficient leverage to start a research program.

Obtaining the scarce resource, money, may be the salient problem in some settings. Particularly in the case of hospitals, third party payers are imposing tight controls on what is to be considered reimbursable. The education of student professionals is one activity coming under scrutiny; many payers now exclude costs associated with student education from reimbursement. While the same stance may hold at the present time with respect to the conduct of research in community hospitals, the situation will change. Former Secretary of HEW, Joseph Califano, in a 1978 policy-setting speech before a national group of researchers, asserted that one of the biggest gaps in health research in our nation is the failure to make appropriate applications of the findings of research to individuals for the improvement of their health. He went on to state as a principle of health research, that "basic research has to be accompanied by vigorous, thoughtful, and where appropriate, interdisciplinary application." He added that there must be a connection "not just between basic and applied research but also among research disciplines."[20]

Six months from the date of the Secretary's historic declaration, a meeting of scientists and researchers from a variety of disciplines was convened by the director of the National Institutes of Health (October 3 and 4, 1978) to critique a set of "planning principles" which are to guide long-range federal support of health research. A number of nurses attended, several of whom testified on behalf of research in nursing. In draft form, at least, the principles explicitly call for research which is supported by federal funds not only to be applied to health care problems, but to require those conducting research and those delivering care to collaborate in the interests of clients/patients. If this principle takes the form of a federal guideline, there is little question that research in health care settings will become an allowable cost.

REFERENCES

1. Conway, M. E. "Organizations, Professional Autonomy and Roles" in Hardy, M. and Conway, M. E., eds. *Role Theory: Perspectives for Health Professionals* (New York: Appleton-Century-Crofts 1978).
2. Scott, R. "Effectiveness of Organizational Effectiveness Studies" in Goodman, P. et al., eds. *New Perspectives in Organizational Effectiveness* (San Francisco: Jossey-Bass 1977).
3. Katz, D. and Kahn, R. *The Social Psychology of Organizations* (New York: John Wiley & Sons 1966) p. 88.
4. Simon, H. "Approaching the Theory of Management" in Koontz, H., ed. *Toward a Unified Theory of Management* (New York: McGraw-Hill Book Co. 1964).
5. Hall, R. H., Haas, J. E. and Johnson, N. J. "Organizational Size, Complexity, and Formalization." *American Sociological Review* 32: (1967) p. 903–912.
6. Perrow, C. *Organizational Analysis: A Sociological View* (Belmont, Calif.: Wadsworth Publishing Co. 1970).
7. Kuhn, A. *The Logic of Social Systems* (San Francisco: Jossey-Bass 1974) p. 5.
8. Ibid.
9. Schrag, C. "Science and the Helping Professions." *Nursing Research* 17: (1968) p. 486–496.
10. Schlotfeldt, R. M. "Nursing Research: Reflection of Values." *Nursing Research* 26: (January–February 1977) p. 4–9.
11. Rogers, M. *Introduction to the Theoretical Basis of Nursing* (Philadelphia: F. A. Davis Co. 1971).
12. Schrag. "Science and the Helping Professions."
13. Argyris, C. and Schon, D. "Theory in Practice" in *Increasing Professional Effectiveness* (San Francisco: Jossey-Bass 1976) p. 4.
14. Cook, T., ed. *Evaluation Studies Review Annual* Vol. 3 (Beverly Hills: Sage Publications 1978) p. 14.
15. Johnson, J. "Effects of Structuring Patients' Expectations on Their Reactions to Threatening Events." *Nursing Research* 21: (1973) p. 499–504.
16. Zimmer, M. "Evaluation Using Patient Health/Wellness Outcome Criterion Variables and Standards" in *Issues in Evaluation Research* (Kansas City: American Nurses Association 1975) p. 62.
17. Horn, B. and Swain, M. A. "An Approach to Development of Criterion Measures for Quality Patient Care" in *Issues in Evaluation Research*, p. 74.
18. Scott. "Effectiveness of Organizational Effectiveness Studies." p. 77.
19. Ibid.
20. Califano, J. "Remarks before the Annual Meeting of the American Federation for Clinical Research." San Francisco, Hilton Hotel, San Francisco, California, April 29, 1978.

GROUP DISCUSSION

Education/Research Component

The following summarizes the group discussions on the education/research component of the nursing administrator's role, which took place at the Boston University School of Nursing conference.

Objectives of Group Discussion

The objectives for these work sessions were:

1. to identify the major nursing issues underlying the education/research component of the nurse administrator's role;
2. to develop a rationale for selecting each issue;
3. to identify the implications of each issue; and
4. to develop educational strategies and/or recommendations for the future.

Four basic assumptions were established initially. Three major issues were then identified and, where appropriate, rationale and implications were articulated. The educational strategies and recommendations for Issue 1 (below) apply to all three issues. The basic assumptions include:

1. Nursing is a science.
2. The practice of nursing is knowledge based.
3. The practice of nursing is research based and must be continually adjusted to take account of new knowledge.
4. The practice of the nurse administrator is administration.

Issue 1: Extent of Research Preparation at the Master's and Doctoral Levels

RATIONALE

Since the role of the nurse administrator involves improving the quality of nursing practice, and since the practice of nursing is both knowledge and research based, preparation in research must be a priority in graduate education programs.

The preparation of nurse administrators with research knowledge and ability will promote parity with medicine and other disciplines and facilitate collegiality and inter- and intradisciplinary research efforts.

IMPLICATIONS

The nurse administrator who has had preparation in research at the graduate level will:

- be more likely to do research;
- be sensitive to the research efforts of staff and colleagues;
- be more likely to apply research findings; and
- have greater potential for doctoral study.

EDUCATIONAL STRATEGY/ RECOMMENDATIONS

Preparation in research will be based on the philosophy of the nursing administration program. The philosophy should be explicit so the student can select the appropriate program.

At the master's level, preparation for conducting research will be included and a thesis will be required. Content in research methodology including the rigor and discipline of research as a thought process is essential. The thesis may be limited to replication of studies and/or original studies in a focused area.

At the doctoral level, preparation to extend knowledge and advance the science of nursing and its practice is the focus. Programs will include extensive exploration and mastery of research methodology as well as cognate areas. The doctoral program will concentrate on meta analysis and theory building to prepare the graduate as a high-level researcher, administrator and consultant. Studies of complex management problems, mergers, organizational design and models for delivery of care are a few of the potential areas for study.

Issue 2: Role of the Nurse Administrator as an Initiator, Facilitator and Utilizer of Nursing Research

RATIONALE

As an *initiator,* the nurse administrator participates in or may originate research. As a *facilitator,* the nurse administrator is responsible for supplying resources and encouraging research to take place. As a *utilizer,* the nurse administrator operationalizes research findings.

The role in each of these areas of nursing research may vary depending upon the setting, the contextual management, organizational control, extent of collegial relationships and the preparation and expectation of nurse administrators. The nurse administrator is expected to maximize research to the greatest extent possible regardless of the setting and situation.

IMPLICATIONS

As an *initiator,* the nurse administrator generates research proposals in nursing practice and nursing administration including such activities as:

- grant writing;
- preservation of data for research;
- organization of studies of both an experimental and nonexperimental nature; and
- initiation of interdisciplinary and intradisciplinary proposals and studies.

As a *facilitator,* the nurse administrator develops an organizational design, including philosophy and structure in which scientific inquiry is the norm rather than the exception. This includes such activities as:

- provision of support for personnel for research including the generation of grant proposals;
- assuring control and intervening for both inter- and intradisciplinary efforts;
- assuring nursing's access to and share of technological resources such as computers;
- provision of time for nursing staff to explore problems needing research as well as for application discussions;
- promotion of placement of grad-

uate students on human subject review committees; and

- promotion or creation of new coalitions of individuals in practice and education to facilitate research and research application.

As a *utilizer*, the nurse administrator evaluates and applies research findings to the practice of nursing. Activities which may be included are:

- keeping up to date with published research;
- evaluation of research findings;
- functioning as part of a network to identify research in process as well as forming coalitions of nurses to promote research utilization;
- promotion of research colloquia to explore research findings and their application;
- modification of administrative and organizational systems to promote utilization of findings; and
- application of change theories in promotion of research findings.

Issue 3: Preparation of the Nurse Administrator for Functioning in Various Settings

To prepare the nurse administrator for functioning in various settings such as university health care centers and community hospitals, it is recommended that:

- doctoral preparation be required for the nurse administrator in university health care centers;
- minimal preparation be the master's degree in nursing administration;
- all master's programs include a functional strand in nursing administration;
- since all master's programs have not had a core of content relating to administration, university faculties assume responsibility to provide continuing education opportunities for nurse administrators currently practicing in the field; and
- attention be directed to preparation of middle managers as well as those at top levels.

Changing Perspectives in Preparing Nurse Administrators

Rebecca Bergman, R.N., Ed.D.
Professor of Nursing
Tel Aviv University
Tel Aviv, Israel

This article offers an international perspective on the educational preparation of the nurse administrator. Professor Bergman submitted the article while a visiting professor at Texas Woman's University in 1978.

—The Editors.

IN SOME COUNTRIES, top nursing positions, such as a director of a school of nursing or a nursing service, are held by physicians or other nonnurses. In other countries, nurses may "have the name but not the game"—they hold the prestigious title but do not wield the real power. This situation has led national and international bodies to emphasize the importance of developing nursing leadership, and assuring nurses their role in administration.

The World Health Organization

(WHO) has emphasized the need for nursing leadership in many documents.[1] The Fourth Expert Committee on Public Health Nursing related the need for personnel to have leadership and support through good nursing service administration in order to do an effective job. Good administration promotes both efficiency—doing the job with economy of time and personnel—and effectiveness—selecting and carrying out activities so as to provide for the greatest possible impact on health behavior.[2]

This stand was reiterated by the Fifth WHO Expert Committee on Nursing in the encouragement of each country to allocate resources to educate nurses at an advanced level to provide future teachers, administrators and expert nursing practitioners. Knowledge needed was cited as: "... the sciences basic to health care and of the social, economic and political forces ... as well as a depth understanding of nursing."[3]

The International Council of Nurses (ICN) recently took a firm stand on the issue of nursing authority. It clearly calls for all types of health care facilities to be directed by qualified directors who are nurses.[4]

The International Labour Organization together with WHO and ICN published a convention report on conditions of work and life of working personnel. Programs of higher nursing education were recommended to prepare nursing personnel for:

> ... the highest responsibilities in direct and supportive nursing care, in the administration of nursing services, in nursing education and in research and development of the field of nursing.[5]

The American Nurses' Association divides nursing administration into three separate levels—executive, middle and first-line—and defines the role of top level nursing administrators in its 1978 statement on the "Roles, Responsibilities and Qualifications for Nurse Administrators."[6]

> The nurse administrator at the executive level is responsible for the nursing department and manages from the perspective of the organization as a whole. . . . The nurse executive ensures that standards of nursing practice are established and implemented so that sound nursing care is provided to consumers. The nurse at the executive level carries the obligation to be a spokesperson for nursing. Such nurses provide leadership and vision in nursing's development and advancement. . . . The nurse executive promotes effective nursing through skillful exercise of the functions of administrator and through broad knowledge of the functions of clinician, researcher and educator. . . . Nurse administrators have as their primary objective the timely achievement of patient care goals. To this end they facilitate nursing research, foster utilization of research findings, and encourage staff development activities which focus on clinical practice. Responsibilities of the nurse administrator include:
>
> 1. Participating in the administration of the total health care agency.
> 2. Determining clinical and administrative goals and directions of the nursing department.
> 3. Devising departmental functions and activities to achieve goals.

4. Acquiring and allocating resources for the determined functions and activities.
5. Evaluating and revising the organizational goals, structures, activities, and resources of the nursing department.
6. Providing leadership in problem solving.
7. Providing leadership in human resources development and personnel management.
8. Providing channels for consumer input into policy development.

All professional nurses are to a degree administrators. Their involvement with and responsibility for administration increases with the scope and complexity of their formal positions within the situational context. As stated by ANA, "nursing administration is the process through which the organized nursing service fulfills its purpose and contributes to the achievement of comprehensive health care."[7] Preparing a nursing care plan, identifying problems in one's nursing practice and seeking solutions for some are all surely part of the "process to achievement of health care." As nurses move up the hierarchical ladder and take on responsibility for guiding, supervising and organizing the work of additional personnel, the scope of their "administration" increases. In addition, as they move from delivery of direct nursing care, where they have the support of an administrative back-up system, to more independent work where they encounter nonroutine situations and have to deal with a greater number of interrelated factors in the system, their administrative role becomes more complex and forms the core rather than the periphery of their nursing practice.

If the role of all professional nurses includes aspects of nursing administration, then all professional nurses must be provided with the appropriate tools for this role in various levels of nursing educational programs. Administration-focused learning experiences must be offered in basic, postbasic, continuing and graduate nursing education programs.

BASIC NURSING EDUCATION

There is a growing trend in RN education, particularly in the generic baccalaureate programs, to provide upper-division experiences in nursing administration. For example, objectives of most such programs state that the graduate should be able to provide nursing leadership at the team leader level. These programs usually include theory and practice of team work in the nursing and interdisciplinary teams, and experience as a nursing team leader in a service setting. In the

In the last few years the nursing schools in Israel have reorganized the hospital-based diploma schools into independent schools offering an RN diploma with some university credits toward a degree in nursing.

last few years the nursing schools in Israel have reorganized the hospital-based diploma schools into independent schools offering an RN diploma with some university credits toward a degree in nursing. In the final six months of these three-year programs, the students elect an internship in the setting of their choice, which includes an upper-division seminar related to that area of practice. One such seminar on nursing administration has the following components:

1. analysis of administration/management problems which the students encounter in their field placement;
2. examination in greater depth of subjects selected by the students such as: orientation of a new staff nurse, team meetings, etc.; and
3. practice in unit management under the preceptorship of the unit head nurse.

POSTBASIC BACCALAUREATE EDUCATION

The Tel Aviv University postbasic baccalaureate program prepares RNs for leadership positions. In order to meet the diverse backgrounds, needs and career objectives of the students, the program includes both elective and required courses. Among the required courses, at least two are directly related to administrative skills. The first of these is a three-semester experience as a change agent.[8] Each student, supported by a tutor, selects a problem from his or her real-life work situation, analyzes its components, examines options for change, develops and implements a plan for change, and evaluates the results of the change. This course is demanding of students and faculty, but has proved to be a most rewarding experience. The other administration requirement, which is interdisciplinary, is concerned with principles of administration.

In relation to electives, many students choose the seminars on nursing administration, on evaluation in nursing or community planning. In addition to the nursing major, students select two minors offered by other departments. The most popular minors are in administration and education.

These specific administration learnings do not, of course, stand alone. They are built upon a base of introductory sociology, anthropology, psychology, research methods, statistics, communication and other courses.

The program described above in the independent schools (with the administration seminar) prepares nurses for unit head-nurse positions. Graduates of the postbasic university program who take electives in administration seminars and the minor in administration should be able to function effectively as supervisors or directors of hospital or community nursing services.

POSTBASIC DIPLOMA COURSES

Some RNs do not wish, or are unable to undertake an academic degree program. Diploma programs are available to these groups, many of whom are already filling administrative positions. The original diploma program was of nine months' duration and focused on nursing administration. It later fused with the postbasic program preparing nurse-teachers, and enabled a healthy exchange of ideas among colleagues.

These courses have now moved from the auspices of the employing agencies into the university in the form of a three-year, one-day-a-week program leading to a university diploma. Most of the courses carry university credits should the student be accepted to a degree program at a later date. These diploma programs are now being offered in three universities and are in great demand.

CONTINUING EDUCATION

Continuing education programs offer another method of preparing nurses for administrative tasks, as well as keeping them up to date. Continuing education refers to learnings which can be undertaken while employed and are related to the present or future position. Some of the organizational patterns are: in-service programs offered by and usually at the place of work; external short-term studies such as workshops or study days; on-going planned part-time out-of-agency programs which may or may not carry formal academic or other credits.

Continuing education should be planned and have long-range objectives. Sporadic offerings may fill an important need in urgent, unexpected situations, but lose much of their value if not integrated into a larger pattern which builds upon the past and forms a base for future learnings.

Examples of justifiable "sporadic" learning in administration may be: the short-term availability of a visitor with specific expertise; the need to quickly prepare nurses for the reorganization of a service; orientation to new health-related laws; and emergency situations such as war or natural calamity.

Long-term continuing education should be planned for a period of several years and be composed of learning blocks that can stand separately (allowing for entrance at various points), but that together synthesize into a comprehensive program.

Continuing education is increasingly receiving formal recognition. Several states in the United States require evidence of continuing education for relicensing. Some courses are recognized as university credit toward a bachelor's or master's degree. In Israel, successful completion of approved courses cumulate into salary benefits.

An exciting example of a comprehensive approach to continuing education is the special department established at the School of Nursing, University of Washington, Seattle.[9] The faculty conducted a survey in order to learn the continuing education needs of nurses in the State of Washington and its neighboring states. This report included recommendations for a mobile unit extension program at various levels (nondegree, bachelor's and master's) as needed in clinical nursing, administration and teaching.

What courses might be desirable for administrators in a continuing education program? The blocks could include learnings for nurses without an academic background such as introduction to psychology, sociology, statistics. Nurses with a first degree or equivalent postbasic study could register for second-level courses such as research methods, biostatistics, epidemiology, communication, group work, interview and foundation of teaching. Upper-division learnings such as systems analysis, labor planning, budgeting, computer science, theories of power, etc., would be appropriate for those at the master level or with sophisticated work experience.

Continuing education programs usually have the advantage of including (1) motivated groups who have clear career goals; (2) an available field from which to draw clinical data and examples; and (3) a setting where learners can test and implement their learnings with the support and guidance of the teachers. Involvement of practicing nurses from different agencies enables an exchange of ideas and experience and often opens the door for cooperation and coordination.

A modest approach for preparing staff nurses for supervision in their public health agency, through continuing education, was described by Littlejohn.[10] The agency selected candidates who had demonstrated their ability in nursing practice and teaching, and who the agency believed had leadership potential.

The first step was to draw up a job description, and then identify what learnings were needed in order to fulfill the desired role. All levels of staff participated in this exercise. Based on the findings, a three-week intensive theoretical and practical program was organized. It included policy and organization of the agency; coordination with other groups; the use of self; and management, education and evaluation. On completion of the program, the new supervisor continued to receive guidance and support in the continuing education program for supervisors.

GRADUATE EDUCATION

Most countries which have university nursing education programs prepare nurse administrators at the master's level. In fact, the early master's degrees almost exclusively offered majors in supervision, administration or teaching. It is only within the last decade that the pendulum has swung from the functional focus to clinical emphasis, because of the felt need to enhance the status and role of clinical nursing. Considerable discussion has

The pendulum has swung from the functional focus to clinical emphasis because of the felt need to enhance the status and role of clinical nursing.

evolved around this move, with some leaders supporting a combined clinical-functional curriculum, and others proposing concentration on one or the other aspect. Blair described the steps taken by the School of Nursing, University of Colorado, for such a new (or new-old) model.[11] They aim to prepare a nurse "with knowledge and skills in nursing research and administration requisite for effective nursing administrative practice in a variety of settings."[12]

The program has three major interlinking components: nursing, administration and research. In the nursing courses students study theories of nursing; analyze various patterns of practice; focus on the application in nursing of theories of power, change, communication, decision making, etc.; as well as the more practical aspects of staffing, budgeting, evaluation and cost analysis. Administration courses are offered in an interdisciplinary setting where major foci are on organizational theories, systems analysis, labor relations, economics, etc.

Research is the third major component. In addition to studying methodology, reviewing and analyzing pertinent studies, the students carry out a research project related to nursing administration.

Many nursing leaders do not agree with Blair. Simms believes nursing administration and clinical specialization are carried out more effectively if each is vested in the role and functions of separate persons who are operationally dependent upon each other for optimizing their roles. In order to provide the environment for the clinical nurse specialist to accomplish patient-centered nursing care, the nurse administrator must understand the purposes and methods of clinical practice. The nursing director must find the personnel and material resources, and maintain the homeostasis between nursing and other developments.[13]

Peterson supports the stand taken by Simms. She believes that nurse administrators need to have skills and methods to enable them to know what is going on, without themselves having a clinical background. Such tools include rounds or field visits, team discussions, meeting with supervisor and head nurse, use of reports and nursing audit.[14]

The philosophy of the Tel Aviv University nursing faculty is that nursing administration is responsible for the provision of clinical nursing care. Therefore, the administrator must have clinical knowledge as well as administrative preparation. Our proposed master's program for nursing administration includes a clinical block (the area is elective) with theory, practicum and individual study. The master's thesis which is concerned with an administrative problem will relate it to the selected clinical area.

A model prepared by Yura et al. shows the components of the nursing leadership process.[15] These form a guide for preparing the leader. The components include scientific knowledge (as related to humans, society, health and nursing); knowledge of the decision-making process, values, the needs and goals of those to be served and/or administered; and comprehension of the situations in which the leadership will be conducted. (See Figure 1.)

Arndt and Huckabay present a detailed program for nursing administration at the graduate level (master's, doctoral). They propose a program to include five "threads," or areas of concentration.[16]

1. "Advanced principles of nursing service administration" is concerned with concepts of administration, planning and policy formation, organization and operation of nursing services, and decision making and problem solving.
2. "Principles of human relations within the health care organization and in the community" includes courses such as personnel administration; group behavior; and theories of learning and instruction applied to patients, students and staff.
3. "Physical environment" relates to patterns of structure, both human and material in health care organizations.
4. "Research" prepares the student to understand, use and conduct scientific investigation.
5. "Nursing specialization," conducted jointly by the university and health care organizations, provides a period of internship

FIGURE 1. COMPONENTS OF THE NURSING LEADERSHIP PROCESS

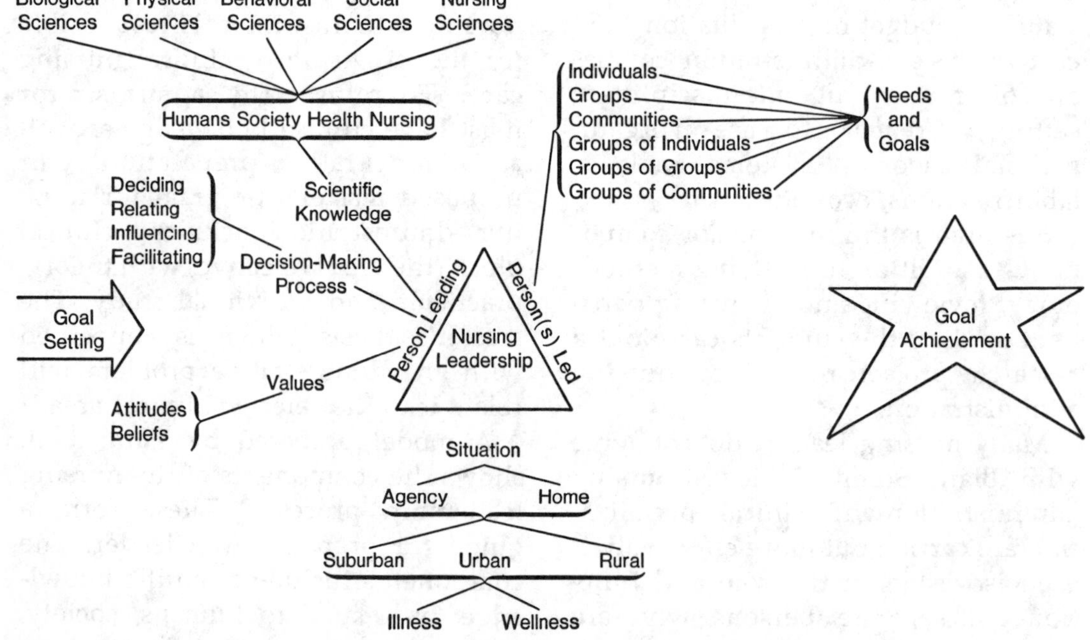

Source: Yura, H. et al. *Nursing Leadership: Theory and Process* (New York: Appleton-Century-Crofts 1976) p. 103. Reprinted by permission.

under the guidance of a preceptor.

Teaching methods for nursing administration are as varied as the subject matter, student characteristics and faculty abilities. Since most of the students in these programs are mature persons, with experience in nursing practice and management, several points should receive special emphasis.

1. Early in the program, the student should be exposed to philosophies, conceptual frameworks and analytical tools.
2. Past and present experiences of students should be used.
3. Students should be involved in setting goals, presenting materials and evaluating.
4. Self-study resources such as libraries, learning modules and programmed learning should be supplied.
5. An arena for group interaction of students and faculty should be provided.
6. Students should be encouraged to apply learning in their practice area, and to be change agents where applicable.

Study with other disciplines is considered of cardinal importance, particularly in preparation for administration. Interdisciplinary person-to-person contact in the learning situation should break down barriers and promote mutual respect and future collaboration. Seminars dealing with health issues and team practice in the field are among the recommended learnings. While fully supporting interdisciplinary education, one must be aware of possible backlash. Nurses and their interests may receive less attention than is their due unless the nursing faculty and students have a firm professional identity. A quota system may take precedence over individual abilities in selection, in order not to overpopulate a program with a single discipline.

EVALUATION

Evaluation is an integral part of all educational endeavors and should be conducted as a continuous process throughout the total program. There are many approaches to evaluation; one is to examine input, process and outcome.

Input

The major components of input in an educational program are students, faculty and facilities.

It is customary to establish criteria for selecting **students.** We need to ask ourselves if these criteria represent the crucial, or even desirable, characteristics needed for nurse administrators. To what degree is age important, and if it is, in what way? Is it better to

It is customary to establish criteria for selecting students. We need to ask ourselves if these criteria represent the crucial, or even desirable, characteristics needed for nurse administrators.

select nurses with experience or those who come to the program without preconceptions? Next, assuming that the criteria are good indicators of successful practice, do we succeed in recruiting candidates who meet these criteria? How do we measure criteria such as intelligence, motivation, quality of past experience?

The second input is **faculty.** What are the educational qualifications of the teachers? Have they kept up with new developments? Do their backgrounds provide the necessary knowledge, attitude and skills for the changing curriculum?

Facilities include the school and the field. Is the library adequate and current? Is modern instructional "hardware" available? Does the field—institutional and community—offer a suitable range of experiences? What is the quality of practice in the agencies? Is there readiness and ability in the field to involve students? Are there logistic problems in utilizing facilities?

Process

Process is the actual "doing" in the program. Are the planned learning experiences carried out? What is the student–teacher ratio? How much independent study is required? How are theory and practice integrated? How are students examined? What is the quality of interpersonal relationships?

Outcome

Outcome, or the "product," is the most crucial of the three elements of evaluation. In evaluating outcome one must return to the curriculum objectives in order to see to what degree they are achieved. Skills and knowledge are reasonably easy to assess; examination of attitudes is more complex. The real crunch comes with on-the-job performance in various situations on completion of the program, and truly objective measures have yet to be devised. Educators tend to believe their responsibility ends with the graduation of the students. We may have to look for long-term measures of applying the learnings, as well as periodically evaluating achievement throughout and on completion of the program.

Cardinal to evaluation is to know what needs to be measured, and to develop criteria and methods for this evaluation—criteria and methods that are essential, clear and as simple as possible. Evaluation sometimes becomes an end in itself and draws upon resources far out of proportion to its value or to the program itself.

MASTER PLAN

One of the issues to be addressed in nursing education is the desirability of determining career plans early. Should young nurses seek their specialization based on available opportunities or should they try to determine their professional future by early preparation for the specific area? Two examples, one from New Zealand and one from the United States, will illustrate.

The New Zealand educational model has five levels and three nursing streams of teaching, clinical practice and management. It allows for career decision in relation to the stream to be made before entering the third level.[17](See Figure 2.)

The Southern Region Education Board Curriculum study proposed a two-dimensional model. The first dimension is level—from vocational (practical) nurse through doctoral preparation. The second dimension is area—clinical practice, research, administration, education and organization. Each level of education leads into a more advanced position. The baccalaureate level permits entry to administration of general hospital units or educational administration of family and patient teaching. The master's program prepares for administration of complex patient units or administration of a nursing education program. The doctoral level develops clinical or educational administrators for leadership in complex programs.[18]

FIGURE 2. NEW ZEALAND EDUCATIONAL MODEL.

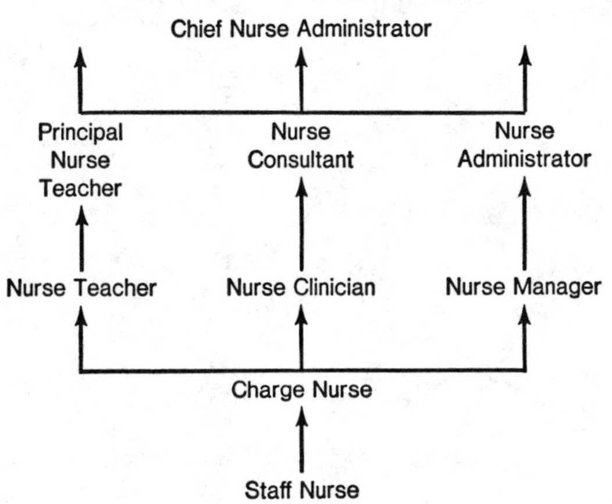

Whether these or other models are selected, one must know where educational programs lead. We have to develop a master plan that will facilitate achievement of career goals with minimal duplication, and that will not exclude transfer into a different stream on completion of supplementary preparation.

Experience and apprenticeship are only complementary to formal preparation for administration. Learning by doing, or even the best apprenticeship program, cannot stand alone in today's sophisticated world of administration. Health care has become big business and needs the knowledge and skills of the highest level if it is to be carried out effectively and efficiently.

Promotion of the health of populations through effective health services is the reason for the existence of nursing and other health professions. Health care depends on human, physical and fiscal resources; and the latter two are made meaningful only by people—the human resource. Nursing needs well-qualified people to administer resources of the nursing component, and to share with other disciplines in designing and implementing total programs. It is up to us, the profession, to assure that nursing leaders are prepared, available and utilized.

REFERENCES

1. World Health Organization. *Public Health Nursing, Fourth Report of the Expert Committee on Nursing* Technical Report Series 167 (Geneva: WHO 1959).
2. Ibid.
3. World Health Organization. *Expert Committee on Nursing* Fifth Report, Techical Report Series 347 (Geneva: WHO 1966).
4. International Council of Nurses, Council of National Representatives. "Statement of Nursing Authority." (Singapore, August 1975).
5. International Labour Organization. *Convention 149 and Recommendation 157 Concerning Employment and Conditions of Work and Life of Nursing Personnel* (Geneva: ILO 1977).
6. American Nurses' Association, Commission on Nursing Services. *Roles, Responsibilities, and Qualifications for Nurse Administrators* (1978) p. 4.
7. Ibid. p. 299.
8. Bergman, R., Greif, L. and Oser, S. "The Practicum—A Learning Experience in Integration and Change." *Journal of Advanced Nursing* 1:3 (June 1976) p. 197–208.
9. University of Washington. *Continuing Nursing Education in Washington State—Expressed Needs* (Seattle: University of Washington 1972).
10. Littlejohn, C. "From Staff Nurse to Supervisor: A Plan of Development." *Nursing Outlook* 24:10 (October 1976) p. 618–621.
11. Blair, E. "Needed: Nursing Administration Leaders." *Nursing Outlook* 24:9 (September 1976) p. 550–554.
12. Ibid. p. 553.
13. Simms, L. "Impact of Patient-Centred Approaches on the Emerging Role of the Clinical Nurse Specialist" in Abdullah, F. et al (eds). *New Directions in Patient-Centred Nursing* (New York: Macmillan 1973).
14. Peterson, G. "Do Nursing Administrators Need Advanced Clinical Preparation?" *American Journal of Nursing* 70:2 (February 1970) p. 297–303.
15. Yura, H., Ozimek, D. and Walsh, M. *Nursing Leadership, Theory and Process* (New York: Appleton-Century-Crofts 1976) p. 103.
16. Arndt, C. and Huckabay, L. *Nursing Administration* (St. Louis: The C.V. Mosby Co. 1975).
17. New Zealand Nurses' Association. *New Directions in Post-Basic Education—Policy Statement on Nursing in New Zealand* (NZNA, September 1976).
18. Hasse, P. "Pathways to Practice—Part II." *American Journal of Nursing* 76:6 (June 1976) p. 850–854.

NURSING SERVICE AND EDUCATION

Uniting Service and Education at Rush-Presbyterian-St. Luke's Medical Center

THE DIVISION OF NURSING AND THE COLLEGE OF NURSING: AN OVERVIEW

THE DIVISION of Nursing at Rush-Presbyterian-St. Luke's Medical Center and at the College of Nursing, Rush University, is organized in a holistic model to build more certainty into the quality of nursing practice, professional education, clinical research and professional consultation. It is assumed, for purposes of this organizational design, that the best-prepared nurses should be arrayed throughout the organization to supply professional leadership at all levels. Thus nurses with advanced preparation are arranged strategically in both horizontal and vertical deployment to facilitate the movement toward excellence in all areas of professional endeavor. Nurses with faculty qualifications function in the entire range of positions from primary nurses to vice president and dean. When this arrangement is combined with decentralization of decision making, the best nursing resources help catalyze all aspects of every nursing program.

Faculty members function as practitioner/teachers. They develop their practice and share it with their students instead of merely visiting units and encroaching on the organized activities of respective clinical areas. Thus faculty members become viable behavioral models of clinical practice, and the discussions in the classrooms become transformed into real phenomena. Furthermore, this arrangement permits faculty members to be in daily contact with puzzling clinical problems. This state of affairs in turn generates increasingly sharp insights into areas most needing clinical research. The presence of so many well-qualified nurses at all levels of professional influence is also a distinct aid in enabling a more rapid dissemination of new research findings and new practice techniques. Additionally, a stronger base for developing more sensitive insight into ethical concern is laid.

The interdisciplinary effort is enriched because nurses with advanced training have more overlap of knowledge systems with colleagues in the other health professions. A more useful metalanguage is operable, and the content of nursing can be woven more expertly into interdisciplinary efforts. Balanced decision making can be made because the training gap between professions tends to be lessened or neutralized. The common respect that is a byproduct of expert power comes into play, professional genuflecting is erased and scientific colleagueship becomes the operating theme.

The presence of a critical mass of nurse faculty members becomes an anchor point around which self-governance for the entire nursing staff can be built. When nurses do become organized in this fashion, it will enable them to become much more responsible for the quality of their clinical practice; to be more alert to the issues of organized care; to be more responsive to the feedback from patients; and to be better able to envisage themselves as vital contributors to the health care endeavor and thus raise self-esteem and desire for career growth.

The assumption of the full professional role is an indication of professional maturity. Disclaimers, who decry its possibility, are holding back the progress of the profession. In those settings where there is movement toward this objective, the response from nurses is positive and productive. The concept is not a unique happening that can be made to work in only relatively few settings. It is a way to support the general development of nursing in all settings in a way that can result in a profession richly endowed with a high degree of clinical capability and greatly enhanced usefulness to patients.

Luther Christman, Ph.D., R.N., F.A.A.N.
Vice President for Nursing Affairs

Rush-Presbyterian-St. Luke's Medical Center
Dean of the College of Nursing
Rush University
Chicago, Illinois

EDUCATION + SERVICE = PROFESSIONAL POWER

Commitment is a lifestyle dominated by a set of values that stimulates the formation and growth of a professional conscience, an inner voice, that guides and monitors behavior. Competence is one of the measureable characteristics of this value system: the level of proficiency is observable because of the wide range of clinical ability. The unfortunate state of disunity between education and service may be a major reason why most nurses have a series of jobs instead of a career and why so few aspire to further preparation. The vigor and energy of a profession are tightly linked to the levels of achieved competence and attained career development. The unnatural separation of education and service may be a prime reason for much of the attenuated commitment evident within the nursing profession.

Role Expression of Knowledge

The amount of scientific knowledge a practitioner possesses is fixed by the individual's level of professional preparation. Clinical behavior is a direct outcome of attained preparation because the predispositions to act in the clinical situation are formed, limited and defined by the quantity of knowledge possessed by each practitioner. Thus the total role expression of knowledge and the quality of individual practice correlates one-to-one with individual knowledge systems. The variation in practice at each level of preparation is most likely a result of the variation in one's ability to apply possessed knowledge in the practice arena. There can be no guarantee that individuals will use the knowledge they possess. However, the structural variables for organizing care are highly influential on the types of expressive behavior. An entirely different outcome is possible where the structure enables synchronized effort in contrast to settings where there are built-in constraints. It follows then that where service and education are not artificially constructed and isolated entities, the full use of knowledge can be mobilized in contradistinction to settings where polarization of these entities hampers the innovative use of knowledge. A heuristic formulation can be made which demonstrates the interrelationship between these factors and the role expression of knowledge. (See Figure 1.)

Many have asserted that the power base of nurses has been weakened unduly because most nurses are women in a society dominated by men. This assertion has only plausible truth. It can be argued that a more basic reason is the limited scientific knowledge system of nurses as contrasted to those of the other major health professionals. Growth in the stature of the

FIGURE 1. FORMULATION OF ROLE EXPRESSION OF KNOWLEDGE

$$\text{Role Expression of Knowledge} = \frac{\left[\left(\sum \begin{array}{l}\text{Theory and}\\ \text{Content of}\\ \text{Science}\\ \text{Possessed*}\end{array}\right)\left(\sum \begin{array}{l}\text{Structural}\\ \text{Constraints**}\end{array}\right)\left(\sum \begin{array}{l}\text{Individual}\\ \text{Clinical}\\ \text{Competence***}\end{array}\right)\left(\sum \begin{array}{l}\text{Range}\\ \text{of}\\ \text{Opportunities}\end{array}\right)\right]}{N}$$

*Cognitive aptitude.

**I.e., matrix vs. hierarchical organization; extent of decentralization of decision making, separation vs. nonseparation of education and service; team nursing vs. primary nursing; and similar entities.

***Sets of nursing skills from traditional to avant-garde.

The full clinical role for any of the clinical professions encompasses the activities generally listed under the concepts of service, education, consultation and research.

nursing profession is more tightly linked to the development of a critical mass of nurses who achieve graduate level preparation (who are thus able to influence care processes through expert power) than it is to increased stature which may be a result of fallout from the women's movement. (Male nurses behave in the same pattern as do female nurses and have similar professional lifestyles. The present form of role induction into the profession overrides sex linkage.) When disparate gaps in levels of scientific knowledge are lessened or eliminated, new relationships take place. An equation may help to visualize these concepts. (See Figure 2.)

Full Clinical Roles

The full clinical role for any of the clinical professions encompasses the activities generally listed under the concepts of service, education, consultation and research. When nurses adopt only one of these subroles and try to force that subrole into a full role activity, a diminution in quality occurs. Furthermore, when large numbers of nurses make this decision, the profession is dichotomized. The growth of the profession is hampered because the growing edge of each group is narrowed and lacks regular stimulation. When the full professional role is achieved, the growing edge has a far different quality. It compares favorably to the progress

FIGURE 2. MODEL FOR GROUP PROFESSIONAL POWER

$$\text{Group Professional Power} = \frac{\left[\left(\sum \begin{array}{l}\text{Educational}\\ \text{Preparation}\end{array}\right)\left(\sum \begin{array}{l}\text{Individual}\\ \text{Clinical}\\ \text{Power}\end{array}\right)\left(\sum \begin{array}{l}\text{Individual}\\ \text{Career}\\ \text{Development}\end{array}\right)\right]}{N}$$

that can be identified in the other major clinical professions where service and education are united.

It is interesting to speculate how much richer the research efforts of nurses might be if the well-prepared faculty members were consistently active in meaningful practice. The essence of research is asking the right questions. If research hypotheses emerged as a byproduct of daily and accountable nurse–patient interaction, research would become more productive and useful to the advancement of practice. One has only to reflect on the enormous preoccupation with the concept of a theory of nursing to draw such a conclusion. The will-o'-the-wisp chase for something that cannot materialize is probably a direct outcome of withdrawal from the empiricism of the real world.

Most of the prominent nurses identified with nursing theory appear to be quite remote from clinical practice, and this may explain their preoccupation with trying to come up with "all or none" interpretations of clinical practice. Expert clinicians must deal with the role expression of knowledge as applied scientists because the fundamental sciences do not change their theory and content with the user. Because nursing practice is an applied science, the integration of service and education into a holistic entity facilitates the use of knowledge in providing nursing care. In addition, role expression is highly modified by the amount of scientific knowledge possessed, by the way the division of labor is organized, by the legal code and by the accountability pattern of the health care delivery system. All of these variables influence the innovative potential and markedly affect contributions to the expert management of health and illness. (See Figure 3.)

The role expression of knowledge can occur in a variety of ways both within and between professions. A consistent expression of scientific knowledge at high levels of usefulness, a continuous acquisition of new knowledge and flexible and imaginative use of knowledge are criteria of excellence in practice. These characteristics are easily developed when a happy marriage of service and education are the basis for the practice under observation.

Role Induction of Students

The role induction of students into the nursing profession is in many

FIGURE 3. A HOLISTIC MODEL FOR INNOVATIVE POTENTIAL

$$\text{Innovative Quotient*} = \frac{\left[\left(\sum \text{Role Expression Potential**}\right)\left(\text{Organizational Design}\right)\left(\text{Attained Group Power}\right)\right]}{N}$$

*Generation and implementation of innovation
**Imaginative application of individual competence

respects as critical to their development as the academic program. Much discussion in the literature has centered around reality shock. A useful hypothesis for investigation is that where students are having their clinical experiences in settings which offer the unification of service and education, they experience much less reality shock. Does the induction process produce qualitative differences in output where studied aloofness, scapegoating, or any other form of less-than-peaceful coexistence is present among nurses, as contrasted to where service and education activities are mutually facilitative? In one setting, the students perform under wraps and must choose sides; in the other, the milieu encourages students to concentrate on learning to be expressive users of knowledge and to emulate skilled nurses functioning as capable applied scientists. Furthermore, the sensitive issues of ethical practice can be examined more thoughtfully where service and education are integral role components.

An Obligation

The full use of knowledge is an obligation each profession owes to the clients it serves. Artificial constraints on full professional competence do a disservice to the public. The academic enterprise cannot remain encapsulated from the empirical utilization of knowledge, and the service system cannot remain insulated from the source of most knowledge, and still produce professional services that will be highly valued by society. The whole issue of the allocation of resources can be more imaginatively addressed when the combined budgets of service and education are employed for this purpose than when each is utilized separately and narrowly. The difference in increasing the professional financial resource for each enclave of nurses so organized is geometrical rather than arithmetical. When the two elements of practice are welded together in a unified whole, a linkage system is in place for clinical access to conduct research; for the rapid dissemination of new knowledge; for the examination of novel and more sophisticated practice issues; and for the growth of a rich media to support more strength and vigor in clinical efforts. In fact, this unification is the absolute basic requisite for the creation of centers of excellence in nursing. No such centers exist in the true sense of the word, but their formation is mandatory to serve as beacons of competent nursing practice to the rest of the field.

The concept of the whole being greater than the sum of its parts has long been accepted in the scientific community. The potential for greatly

---

The potential for greatly enhancing the cognitive and behavioral patterns of nurses by the equation that education and service equals professional power is full of promise.

---

enhancing the cognitive and behavioral patterns of nurses by the equation that education and service equals professional power is so full of promise that considerable effort should be used to bring about full development of its implications. Some disruptions in present lifestyles, established career patterns and organized groups will occur. However, the benefits to patients, the increased social value of the profession and the self-actualization of each nurse have so much promise that these gains far outweigh the status quo rewards presently offered. At this time in the development of the profession, the burden of proof may well lie with those who are attempting to develop the profession holistically. However, the odds would seem to favor these group efforts over those that insist on fragmentation. The catalytic force developed by the unifiers will fuel the profession.

Luther Christman, Ph.D., R.N., F.A.A.N.
Vice President for Nursing Affairs
Rush-Presbyterian-St. Luke's Medical Center
Dean of the College of Nursing
Rush University
Chicago, Illinois

STAFF NURSES ACHIEVE ROLE SATISFACTION WITH HELP OF A PRACTITIONER/TEACHER

A nursing care delivery system that combines education and service provides an environment in which staff nurses are consistently stimulated to develop their individual professional roles. The full expression of these roles should facilitate nursing actions in the areas of service, education, consultation and research. The stimulus to grow comes from all participants in the system, including practitioner/teachers, students and fellow staff nurses who possess varying degrees of education and experience. Each of these practice at different levels in a continuum of nursing expertise, thus always providing ideal behavioral models for the newer members of the profession and continually spreading fresh ideas to higher levels of conceptualization as nurses rise in the career ladder. A separation of service and education creates a gap in this continuum, leaving the student with reality shock, the staff nurse without adequate and easily accessible education (or the motivation to seek it) and the teacher with abstract, rather than reality-based, educational offerings. The ultimate effect of this gap is to hinder the development of the nursing profession.

When students enter the nursing profession, particularly with baccalaureate preparation, a concept that permeates all of the teachings is that education and service are interdependent, unable to exist autonomously without stagnation and regression. Education must be continual, or the resultant low quality service will meet the needs and demands of patients poorly. Conversely, service must consistently provide for application and testing of nursing educational principles to keep what is being learned innovative and useful to the provider of this service of nursing. An educational institution may fall short in providing for adequate role induction of students into the profession if it is not able to support this theoretical framework in the clinical setting.

The Role of Clinical Settings

Often, faculty members are teaching students in facilities that are committed primarily to service. As visitors, the instructors and students have only limited and temporary influence on the quality of clinical nursing practice in these agencies. The setting not infrequently demonstrates to nursing students that the role of the staff nurse is that of providing for patients in a time-oriented, task-specific daily routine, asked only to harmoniously coexist with visiting students and faculty, not to encourage or facilitate interactions on a collaborative basis. This sets up a state of role conflict for students, who wish to become fully role-developed, practicing RNs in the way they are being taught to perform. They fear becoming apathetic, incomplete nurses, with a future that appears destined to occur in care facilities committed primarily to service which are not additionally concerned with the professional development of staff nurses' potential as high quality care providers.

Staff nurses, in a system such as this, are not stimulated to question daily practice, to seek answers and to further education, nor are they rewarded adequately for these efforts. Most staff nurses inevitably become stagnant and indoctrinated with outdated nursing practices; thus they are unreceptive to the brief and distant exposure to the teachings of visiting faculty. Too many nursing service administrators and nursing educators do not yet view the components of service and education as being crucial to the full expression of the nursing role. This is further evidence of the long-standing effects this insulation from each other has had on the profession.

Consistent Interaction

Rush-Presbyterian-St. Luke's Medical Center fosters consistent interaction of nurses with students and faculty in a system that facilitates role development, expression and satisfaction in all areas of service, education, consultation and research. Staff nurses take their place in the continuum as orientees, with initial exposure to both experienced staff nurses (as preceptor/educators) and to the already familiar instructor figures (clinical practitioner/teachers), each particularly skilled in specific areas of nursing practice. The transition from student to graduate to staff nurse is eased by the support and guidance of these individuals, often reducing reality shock and expediting induction of the student into the nursing profession. As orientees evolve into beginning primary nurses, the application of the learned interdependence of education and service can be observed: orientees focus on attainment and improvement of technical skills which are necessary to achieve competency and to correlate these skills with theory to provide quality care. The preceptor/preceptee relationship continues, with the former acting as support provider, behavioral model and resource person.

Primary nurses also quickly seek to learn from the education and experience of assistant head nurses, head nurses and practitioner/teachers as resources in planning for particularly complex nursing problems. Soon functioning as independent practitioners, primary nurses begin to share their patients with nursing students with the guidance and evaluation of practitioner/teachers. This stimulates an exchange of some new and innovative ideas of students with the individualized, sensitive knowledge of primary nurses in the mutual planning, implementation and evaluation of patient care. The staff nurse in this situation identifies both as a fellow learner with the student and as a fellow educator with the teacher. Ultimately the staff nurse functions as a teaching assistant to the practitioner/teacher, who serves as the pacemaker for nursing practice. Through this continued exposure to students, who are usually avidly eager to learn, and to the practitioner/teachers, who are usually eager to share their knowledge, staff nurses are stimulated to seek education and to question practices through increasingly more formalized research efforts. In addition to recognizing the personal satisfaction of reaching developmental goals, the medical center formally recognizes growth through staff nurses' levels of practice credentials. When nurses function in the primary nursing format they consistently interact with other health professionals in an interdependent fashion to provide health care. The primary nurse and the primary physician care for the total patient, coordinating contributions of physician specialists, pharmacists, dieticians and other consultants for individual aspects of care. When nurses are able to fully develop all aspects of their professional role and to become accountable for its expression, they are able to act as clinical partners with physicians in providing patient care. They are increasingly relied on by more physicians as invaluable colleagues.

Allowing education to remain severed from service in the delivery of nursing care produces RNs with incomplete role development, which blossoms into role dissatisfaction, with resultant untimely, poor quality care and a predictable exodus of potentially excellent nurses from the profession. Reuniting the two parts of a whole will produce satisfied and continually growing nurses who provide excellent nursing care. This supports the development of a strong nursing profession. More nursing educators and nursing service admin-

More nursing educators and nursing service administrators must recognize their positions as controllers of the destiny of the nursing profession.

istrators must recognize their positions as controllers of the destiny of the nursing profession. They must unite in the common goal of assuring its growth to the highest possible perfection by implementing the union of service and education in all levels of nursing practice throughout the continuum, from the nursing student to the staff nurse, to the practitioner/teacher and to the administrator/educator.

Mary L. Knue, R.N., B.S.N.
Staff Nurse
Special Care Nursery
Department of Ob/Gyn Nursing
Rush-Presbyterian-St. Luke's Medical Center
Chicago, Illinois

A GROWING EDGE FOR STAFF NURSES

Nursing education began within the clinical practice of nursing. Nurses were educated and trained within the institution by other nurses, by learning theory and by practicing skills in the actual clinical setting. As institutions of higher learning developed nursing programs, nursing education was gradually pulled away from hospital settings and placed on campuses. Hence, a diminution of the clinical facet of nursing education took place—an undesirable hindrance to the conceptualization and development of academic preparation. The further the separation of education and practice, the more dubious became the quality of the clinical orientation of the students. The major contributors to nursing education became pure academicians shed of their clinical role. In the progressive system at Rush, however, there is an attempt to restore the full complement of all variables to the process of nursing education. Those primarily responsible for the supervision and education of students are also responsible for the professional development and growth of the staff and for the development of clinical research. All activities become a group effort, working for both students and staff. The group includes staff nurses and students, a practitioner/teacher and the unit leader.

The Unit Leader

The managerial "head" for the unit is the unit leader. Like the head nurse, a unit leader is responsible for the functioning of the unit, which includes administrative responsibilities for the direction of clinical nursing activities in the patient care area, and for caring for assigned primary patients. Unlike the head nurse, however, the qualifications for the position encompass a broader spectrum. The unit leader possesses a minimum of a master's degree in nursing and functions as a participating member of the faculty of Rush University College of Nursing. In this way, the clinical unit is tied directly to academia. The unit leader keeps the staff informed of educational activities available at the College and is more education and research oriented in the approach to the nursing enterprise on the unit. A major focus is on the continuing education of staff nurses through inservice offerings targeted at specific identified needs. As an active member of the total educational process, the unit leader attains a wider perspective in dealing with the unit and is a teacher as well as an administrator and behavioral model.

The general agreement of RNs on my particular unit (who have worked under both a head nurse and later under a unit leader) seems to support the opinion that educational development on the unit is more emphasized when a unit leader is in place. Being so closely tied to the College provides additional avenues for exploration of options in educational development for staff nurses. The head nurse was often more available for immediate consultation, however, because the responsibility was limited only to the unit.

The unit leader, then, is active in a much broader range of endeavor, including the educational system as well as the clinical setting. Expectations of the unit leader include: supervising and directing clinical nursing activities and educational development of nursing staff; participating in formal student education, in administrative responsibilities to the unit and in departmental activities; and supporting ongoing research. This develops the role into a widely diversified one, which in turn directly affects the staff nurse on the unit and the overall philosophy under which that unit functions.

Practitioner/Teacher

The term practitioner/teacher is almost self-explanatory. Not only does this position include a teaching role on the faculty of Rush University, but it also involves being a unit-based, responsible practitioner. The staff of the unit become familiar with this person first as a fellow patient care giver, who selects primary patients, plans and implements their care and occasionally rotates to other shifts. This encourages and develops a collegiate relationship. As the practitioner/teachers become more familiar with the floor and the staff, they begin to function increasingly as resource staff, presenting inservice sessions, helping to identify and remedy shortfalls in practice, being there to answer questions and serving as consultants to practice.

On my unit this is well exemplified. The staff nurses believe they can rely on the two practitioner/teachers, not only as excellent resource persons who are readily available, but also as patient care givers, committed to meeting patient needs with the same concern displayed by staff nurses. The intermeshing of roles makes for an interesting, yet very comfortable, peer–teacher relationship. The practitioner/teacher functions not merely as a representative of Rush University, but more as a contributing member of the unit. This establishes a considerably different professional atmosphere than the traditional behavior of the clinical instructor on a unit when service and education are not thus united. The traditional instructor enters the unit after little or no contact with the patients and nurses on that unit and attempts to construct a cohesive staff–student relationship that is frequently superficial at best. As a result, students often conclude that they are in the way or are bothersome to the staff nurses.

It is easy to see, with the practitioner/teacher–staff relationship already established, how much smoother the accommodation to students is when they are on the unit. The practitioner/teacher and staff are coworkers, the working relationship has already been tested and, if it is a good one, the students are more likely to be welcomed by the staff. The middleman needed for enhancing staff–student relationships is already solidly oriented to, and accepted on, the unit.

This is not to say that some of the long-standing friction which exists between staff and students in traditional schools of nursing does not exist in this system. Staff nurses are heard to comment that they feel watched and criticized by students, that students are often given priority of general areas on the unit (i.e., keeping staff out of conference rooms during lengthy postconference sessions) and that they are annoyed and frustrated by the limited skill levels which students bring to the unit. However, in the traditional situation of clinical orientation of students, the staff nurses have only a visiting instructor from a specific college with whom to discuss these concerns; in this system, they are able to deal with a person they already know and with whom they have worked. Staff nurses are able to communicate more freely the tensions and uneasiness they have and can consequently effect a means of bettering the milieu for all who are involved. Thus staff nurses, practitioner/teachers and students work together for the good of the unit as a whole, as opposed to each role functioning separately and in disjunction from each other in an atmosphere of suspicion and covert conflict.

Staff Nurses

Not only is the practitioner/teacher involved in student education, but staff nurses have a good deal of influence on many areas of the clinical orientation. Students are assigned patients, and patients have primary nurses responsible for their individual care. This immediately establishes for the student a reliable reference source regarding the care of each patient—someone who is familiar with the patient's hospitalization, problems and idiosyncracies, and someone who can answer questions in a knowledgeable manner regarding care and progress of patients. While working with patients, students are responsible for contributing to the nursing care plans. Staff nurses offer feedback to the educational process by completing simple evaluation forms which are given to the practitioner and shared with each student. Contrast this with the traditional educational format, where students must glean information about patients solely from sporadically available charts; where no one person is responsible for planning care (which often results in a lack or absence of continuity in plans); and where, when student input is made, there is seldom any feedback at all (leaving students to wonder if the suggestions are even read, let alone implemented). In essence our system gives students a behavioral model in a primary nurse as well as a practitioner/teacher; gives them source of reference for patient care; sets expectations for input into the plan of care; provides feedback from faculty and staff; and essentially breaks down the "us versus them" atmosphere that frequently is caused by little or no interaction between staff and students in the conventional orientation to clinical practice. The quality of clinical practice is thus not only influenced by, but also influences, nursing education.

ENLARGED ROLE

An enlarged role for the staff nurse in relation to nursing education at Rush is that of the teaching assistant. Although teaching assistants are held accountable for only a minimal amount of student observation, the role responsibility primarily involves helping in the choice of patients for weekly assignment according to the syllabus of courses being followed in the College. Every specific patient choice is correlated with material being covered in lectures and seminars throughout the week, as opposed to the random patient selection and assignment that may occur in other settings. Nursing theory is read, heard, learned and practiced at the same time.

Nursing theory is read, heard, learned and practiced at the same time.

One of the most important contributions made by teaching assistants is attendance at student experience postconferences. It is surprising and satisfying to note how much input a staff nurse can have by attending just a few of these conferences. The students listen intently to comments, to suggestions and to experienced advice. Conversely, the staff nurse better understands both the students' levels of anxiety when coming to the unit and their personal concerns regarding nursing care in general. Staff and students are mutually enlightened by the professional exchange of observations.

REALITY COMPARISON

A staff nurse sitting in on a postconference personifies reality. The input that is offered examines educational expectations against practical possibilities and contrasts abstract ideals with authentic reality.

One particular example of this occurred not long ago on our unit. A student inadvertently overheard a nurse assert that her job becomes routine. This statement was shared with the rest of the student group, and some apprehensions were expressed about this comment. The practitioner/teacher instructed the students to observe a staff nurse the next day and see what about the job appeared to be routine. Impressions and comments were to be taken to the postconference and discussed. A teaching assistant from the unit was present. Most of the students said they had concluded that what they observed did not seem routine. The teaching assistant was asked for input and helped students to explore alternatives in behavior.

Nursing can become routine. Just as many other jobs, no matter how exciting and innovative, there are tasks which must be done every day and which are less fulfilling than one would desire. Each individual has the responsibility to direct the creativity and the energy it takes to make a job exciting. That supervision for those decisions lies within the individual, in whatever direction is chosen. Nursing is a very diverse field; energies can be directed, and personal fulfillment and intellectual stimulus achieved, in many ways. It is up to the individual to take the initiative to make clinical practice exciting instead of mundane.

Communicating this concept to the students was an important part of their education. Perhaps by having participated in this session, one step in the socialization into clinical practice will be smoother. The students were rapt with attention; the staff nurse was certain she was sharing with them a perspective she wished had been shared with her before entering a full-time clinical position. The session not only opened gates of communication, but also served to bring the students closer to existing reality. The staff nurse had a valuable contribution to make to the educational process, and her contribution was appreciated and utilized by the students.

Education and Clinical Practice Integrated

Only in a primary nursing setting where accountability and autonomy are now encouraged can this blend between education and clinical practice be achieved. The fine meshing of communication among staff, students, unit leaders and practitioner/teachers cannot exist in a fragmented setting that lacks continuity and cohesiveness of nursing efforts. Students in traditional schools of nursing function as primary nurses for their assigned patients—identifying needs, planning care, performing all necessary tasks for the patient. What better behavioral model is there than a staff nurse who also functions as a primary nurse—one who also develops a plan of care and who performs tasks necessary for the welfare of patients? Students learn not only from what they are taught in the classroom, but also from invaluable input on the unit from staff members. Staff members, in turn, benefit from continual educational input into their own practice. This in turn increases both quality and creativity in patient care. Patient care is benefited by more accurate clinical orientation of students and by more creative care planning by nurses who have close available resource persons and who are subject to continual educational stimulus.

The integration of education and clinical practice in this medical center directly affects and enriches the role of staff nurse. It provides opportunities for growth not only within the hospital itself, but also within the programs of the university. The resources available to the staff nurse are jointly provided by the university and the clinical setting, successfully integrating education with practice, as well as encouraging further personal and professional growth of each individual nurse.

Every system has shortcomings. At Rush there are areas requiring further study that will cause revision of goals. This system, however, is a working model of a positive interrelationship between nursing service and education. The end result becomes a cohesive process of nursing education, teaching and practice. Each draws from and enhances the other to benefit and increase the quality of patient care and to better the individual nurse (as a person and as a member of a health profession, a participant on a health care team and a contributor to the development of the profession as a whole). When practice and education become unified, a holistic approach is created which is self-perpetuating and self-rewarding.

Ann Mowry, R.N.
Staff Nurse
Department of Medical Nursing
Rush-Presbyterian-St. Luke's Medical Center
Chicago, Illinois

A UNIFIED ROLE FOR NURSING

The nursing profession is striving to develop a unified theory for practice. Many models constructed in an attempt to arrive at theory are based on a holistic approach. The basis for such an approach is to consider the individual as a physiological, psychological and social being in continuous interaction with the environment. At the same time that nursing labors over holistic concepts for patient care, it continues to separate master's-prepared nurses into exclusive categories of either service or education. If the movement toward holism is viewed as beneficial for the individual as a patient, why does nursing withhold the same benefit for itself? How can nursing expect to achieve a theory based on a holistic approach if it espouses a separatist approach between education and service at the same time?

Many master's-prepared nurses have skills in education, clinical practice, research and consultation. Why then are they often expected to express a mutually exclusive role of service or education? Is it reasonable to expect nurses to teach current practice issues if they are not active in clinical practice? Is it reasonable to expect nurses to test out new theories or research findings in clinical situations without involvement in nursing academics? The longer nursing avoids an integrated role, the longer its professional environment will be deprived of all its resources.

The Role of Practitioner/Teachers

The administrative philosophy at Rush-Presbyterian-St. Luke's Medical Center supports the belief in an integrated nursing role by employing practitioner/teachers. A practitioner/teacher is a master's-prepared nurse who has responsibilities in both nursing education and clinical practice. Research and consultation are encouraged and are expected to occur as an outgrowth of this role. Each is assigned to a specific patient care unit for clinical practice in addition to having a faculty appointment. The most difficult period of role adjustment occurs in the beginning when the new practitioner/teacher is achieving a balance between the practice role and educational responsibilities. A contributing factor to this adjustment lies in the socialization process of a nurse. Nursing education often tends to socialize graduate nurses into single role expression similar to that of the educators themselves, necessitating a period of professional readjustment into the integrated role. However, in the Medical Center, role adjustment is facilitated by 150 other practitioner/teachers.

Nursing education often tends to socialize graduate nurses into single role expression similar to that of the educators themselves, necessitating a period of professional readjustment into the integrated role.

One Medical Center unit within the Department of Community Health Nursing is the Rush Home Health Service (RHHS), a hospital-based home care agency providing skilled nursing services to homebound clients. Approximately one third of the RHHS staff are practitioner/teachers, two of whom have line positions. Those in line positions are designated unit leaders who manage and coordinate the daily activities of the agency to meet organizational objectives. They are ultimately responsible for the care delivered to RHHS patients. Their administrative role is in addition to faculty and practice responsibilities. However, in order to adjust for this additional responsibility, the faculty and practice components are reduced. In contrast to more traditional home care agencies, RHHS utilizes master's-prepared nurses in other than supervisory roles and does not rely on visiting faculty for student clinical experience. Therefore RHHS is administered and staffed by active faculty members with primary care responsibilities, in conjunction with staff nurses and home health aides.

The integrated role of the practitioner/teacher within RHHS is complex, containing several components. The most appropriate way to discuss role expression in this setting is to describe the most common activities of the role: providing primary nursing care to a caseload of patients, teaching students, collaborating and consulting on patient care issues and contributing to decisions regarding agency policy.

AS PRIMARY NURSE AND TEACHER

Practitioner/teachers are active primary nurses to RHHS patients. The number of patients carried by each is individualized and variable. Caseloads are determined by the number of patients needed for student experiences, other academic and professional commitments and individual expertise. This role creates a unique situation which is different from other traditional home care agencies. Instructors at other agencies are often visitors and sometimes need to borrow patients from staff nurses to provide student clinical experience. Often the student learns from the staff nurse who knows the patient's care needs. At RHHS, however, patients of practitioner/teachers are shared with students; hence learning and/or role modeling occur directly from the instructor, who is capable of providing clinical experience which is closely correlated with course objectives. This situation is more intimate and comfortable for the patient because the student can be viewed as an extension of an already established nurse–patient relationship.

Involvement in both clinical practice and academics has advantages in keeping practitioner/teachers current in determining areas in need of research, which is expected to occur as an outgrowth of the integrated role. Two separate research projects are presently being conducted by practitioner/teachers at RHHS. One is a clinical research project studying long-term medication compliance in the elderly. The other is an administrative research project to develop a management information system through the collaborative efforts of RHHS, the Quality Assurance Department and Medicus Systems Corporation.

Not all practitioner/teachers are skilled or interested in designing and conducting a research project. Moreover, availability of time due to other role demands and professional commitments precludes research involvement. Therefore while the role of nurse researcher is encouraged, it is elective rather than mandatory.

AS NURSING CONSULTANTS

Historically, nurses have not had to concern themselves with cost effectiveness in health care delivery because nursing services were folded into the price of a hospital bed. However, with rapid inflation in health care costs, many health care disciplines and consumers are concerned and are striving to provide quality care at the most reasonable price.

The cost of nursing services to home care patients at RHHS is obvious because it is separate from hospital costs. Practitioner/teachers, nursing staff and nursing students are cognizant of the cost of their professional nursing services. This knowledge serves to motivate nurses to provide the best quality of care available.

Often this motivation becomes evident during weekly staff meetings where collaboration and consultation occur freely between nurses and other health care professionals. A climate of professionalism exists in that each member, regardless of educational background, shares special areas of knowledge, interest and/or expertise that apply to patients discussed as a means to provide quality care. It is in this setting that practitioner/teachers express their role as consultants because they are often requested to advise staff or to conduct a home visit to offer their expertise in resolving a patient care problem.

Nursing students benefit from this professional experience through active participation and learn the value of nursing consultation and collaboration with other health care professionals. Such meetings also provide students with knowledge of community and professional resources.

AS DECISION MAKERS

The practitioner/teachers based at RHHS not only practice and teach at the agency but also have an investment in its present and future operations. Since they express their professional role in this setting, there is a commitment to maintain or improve the environment to meet the needs of patients, employees and students. This commitment is evidenced by their serving as members with staff nurses on standing RHHS policy committees. Chairpersons are elected by their respective committee members from either professional level. Committee participation emphasizes a member's contributions to decisions affecting RHHS, its patients and employees.

Each committee is in need of both levels of nursing members to ensure equal representation prior to obtaining approval from leadership. Since policies are decided in a democratic manner, there is virtually no dissension from either group when it is time for implementation.

Practitioner/teachers, as part of the entire medical center and of the university, also participate on larger, more complex medical center and/or university committees. This involvement serves to integrate their role into the institutional framework, provides an opportunity for exchange of knowledge with other practitioner/teachers and incorporates clinical knowledge into university decisions.

The work environment of those who are active in service, education, research and consultation can be both stimulating and motivating. However, the diverse role components can make choices difficult. For example, conflict arises when a practitioner/teacher's patient requires an immediate nursing assessment and there are students in the clinical area. A dichotomy then results between the patient's needs and the students' learning experiences. Solutions are not readily available in this new role, and there is no general rule on how to prioritize and manage these situations.

Commitment to a Unified Role

In summary, the integrated practitioner/teacher role is variable and complex because it is not limited to any one specific area of expression. It is more reasonable to assume teachers of nursing to be expert if they are also in active practice. Concomitantly, it is more reasonable to assume practitioners of nursing have current theoretical knowledge if they are academically involved. Since the nursing profession is striving to develop a unified theory for practice, a commitment to provide a unified role for nursing (which encompasses service, education, research and consultation) should be compatible. In this manner, nursing can more rapidly advance because it is utilizing all of its professional resources.

Sandi Spilotro, R.N., M.P.H.
Practitioner/Teacher
College of Nursing
Rush-Presbyterian-St. Luke's Medical Center
Chicago, Illinois

GETTING IT TOGETHER: THE PRACTITIONER/TEACHER

The student said to the head nurse, "I'd like to have a patient conference on Mr. Kash. When would be a good time?" With determination in her voice, the head nurse responded, "My dear, we don't *have* patient care conferences here!" Situations similar to this have occurred to all of us at one time or another. But this need not occur! The traditional problem of those in service and those in education being at odds with one another has been resolved at Rush through implementation of the practitioner/teacher model.

Practitioner/teachers are faculty members with master's or doctoral degrees who actively effect quality patient care in the clinical and classroom settings through an integrated role as clinician, educator, consultant and researcher. This complex yet challenging role is made possible by an organizational matrix model designed to integrate all aspects of nursing. The matrix model provides a means of organizing human resources in a way that permits the optimum usefulness of the full content of the professional role.

At Rush, every nurse from the vice president of nursing to the staff nurse is actively involved in both patient care and nursing education.

Primary Functions

The primary function of the practitioner/teacher position is to weld, in a highly coordinated and visible fashion, all the activities that are major influences on health care and professional education. Initially, the practitioner/teacher position may appear to be two full-time jobs. However, economy of effort is inherent in this holistic role. Clinical and educational activities encompassing the aspects of research and consultation are performed simultaneously in one environment.

CLINICAL PRACTICE

First and foremost, clinical practice is essential to the viability of the practitioner/teacher position. Because practitioner/teachers are members of the nursing staff of a specific unit, they are an integral part of that unit and therefore have a built-in arena for practice, education, consultation and research.

Because practitioner/teachers are members of the nursing staff of a specific unit, they are an integral part of that unit.

A myriad of possibilities exists for the ways in which practitioner/teachers carry out their clinical endeavors. They may provide patient care as primary nurses and at the same time work closely with the staff members to develop each individual's nursing practice. As consultants, practitioner/teachers utilize their expanded knowledge base and advanced skills. They do so by assisting staff nurses to develop creative solutions to puzzling, difficult patient care situations and by collaborating with members of other health professions on health care issues and patient care problems. Practitioner/teachers are also members of the unit leadership group, the policy-making body for the clinical area. Thus in an administrative capacity they take part in shaping unit policy and patient care standards. Often practitioner/teachers encounter intriguing situations which pose questions for investigation. The flexibility of the role allows individuals to pursue clinical problems in depth through research studies. As a result, practitioner/teachers can disseminate their findings and apply them to patient care immediately, eliminating the usual time lag imposed by formal presentation.

EDUCATION

Perhaps the most personally appealing advantage of the practitioner/teacher position is that the faculty member does not have to forego clinical practice in order to teach. The pragmatic advantages of combining clinical practice and education are many. For example, because the practitioner/teacher knows the patients on the unit well, selection of appropriate student assignments and preparation for student clinical practicum are expedited. Faculty members need not spend hours leafing through charts nor additional time establishing rapport with the patients because most assignments are from their primary patient caseload. When educational responsibilities include lectures or seminars, practitioner/teachers have current material readily available from their varied clinical experiences. By being active in the clinical area, the practitioner/teacher can be more certain that teaching content is up-to-date.

As an integral staff member, the practitioner/teacher bridges the gap between staff members and students. This creates a unique educational environment for student experiences. Students are welcomed on the unit, as opposed to being caught in the crossfire commonly seen in traditional educational settings where student and teacher invade the territory of the nursing staff and are viewed as "outsiders" or "guests." In the integrated health care system, the nursing staff is actively involved in the educational effort in the roles of clinical teaching assistants who are familiar with both the curriculum and the student objectives.

Nursing students are educated from a rich vantage point, that of having a teacher who is a behavioral model. Working side-by-side with practitioner/teachers, students learn to provide quality patient care. They also have the opportunity to observe firsthand appropriate professional behavior and the relationship of parity among practitioner/teachers, physicians and other health team members who combine their skills in caring for patients. This method of education, which incorporates students as part of the team, prevents them from remaining peripheral to actual nursing situations. This helps to decrease the "reality shock" often seen as students become staff nurses.

The educational focus of the practitioner/teacher is not limited to the boundaries of formal education of students. At Rush staff nurses are also offered the stimulation and challenge of the educational milieu. Practitioner/teachers act as consultants to individual nurses and take an active part in conferences and inservice activities where staff members learn to apply educational principles and research findings to patient care.

Advantages

The most significant advantage of the practitioner/teacher role, as mentioned earlier, is the fact that faculty members do not have to forego clinical practice in order to teach. Therefore the nurses who are the best educated and most qualified both teach and provide patient care.

Presently at Rush there are over 150 practitioner/teachers with multiple areas of expertise and diversity of talent. They create a milieu of professional excellence and constant interchange, adding to individual and group stimulation. This allows faculty members to tap knowledgeable resources for almost any type of patient care questions in an educational or a research situation. They can draw on one another's expertise and complement each other's strengths. The "critical mass" of faculty members allows each person to have the opportunity to pursue all aspects of the role in varying degrees over time.

Reasonable tradeoffs, which permit effective utilization of time and resources, are made among practitioner/teachers so that each individual may experience professional achievement and satisfaction while meeting organizational goals. Lastly, because the organization is composed of interdependent relationships rather than a rigid hierarchical structure, practitioner/teachers have independence in decision making and the freedom to introduce change.

Limitations

It would be unrealistic to expect that a position which combines all aspects of nursing would be without its limitations. The limitations, however, are not inherent in the role itself but are rather a result of lack of preparation for it. There are very few behavioral models for the faculty qualified person who wishes to exercise the full professional role. This causes a state of uneasiness for anyone who enters a practitioner/teacher position because it has not been part of experiential learning.

Most nurses have some false starts before they are able to internalize the role. With so many diverse possibilities for professional expression, one may get caught up in the whirlwind of activity. Each faculty member may feel a stimulus overload and a pull in many directions. This forces each practitioner/teacher to analyze individual goals and objectives.

Promise for the Future

Nurses who seek practitioner/teacher positions find themselves in a challenging, dynamic enterprise. A position that combines education and practice is demanding and time consuming, but one must recognize that time and energy are required for any professional role. Everyone must make decisions which determine ultimate self-development. The individual who selects the practitioner/teacher role must be able to critically examine and evaluate multiple options and set discriminate priorities. Skills in negotiation, communication and adherence to one's established priorities are qualities which are vital to satisfaction in the practitioner/teacher role. The person who is self-directed and whose productivity and creativity are aroused by multiple opportunities will find a great deal of satisfaction in the practitioner/teacher position.

Expressing the full professional role has become a reality for practitioner/teachers at Rush. The satisfaction and fulfillment experienced by professionals who can influence patient care through combining education and practice is virtually limitless. The full development of the potential of the role holds promise for the growth of the power and influence of the nursing profession.

The satisfaction and fulfillment experienced by professionals who can influence patient care through combining education and practice is virtually limitless.

Margaret Hansen, R.N., M.S.
Teacher/Practitioner
Surgical and Operating Room Nursing
Rush-Presbyterian-St. Luke's Medical Center
Chicago, Illinois

SERVICE AND EDUCATION UNITED IN THE CHAIRPERSON ROLE

Practice, education, research and administration are the key ingredients for professional power in nursing. Development of expertise in these basic components of nursing practice is the responsibility of all nurses, but the major accountability for the guidance and direction of the nursing profession resides in nurses who have been prepared at the doctoral level. Although this group has increased significantly in number over the past decade, the total cadre of nurses with earned doctoral degrees is still less than one percent of the total nursing profession. Nurses prepared at this highest level of education can indeed enhance the credibility of nurses throughout the health care system because their credentials are comparable to other health experts in the health care delivery system. Their advanced knowledge and expertise is regarded as a resource for power and a key to excellence in service and education.

A basic problem that faces the nursing profession is the unwillingness of nurses to address themselves to the lack of doctorally prepared nurses within nursing. All too often nurses bemoan their lack of professional nursing power and attribute the cause to forces external to the nursing profession. Although there are many individuals within nursing who believe that nursing power will automatically increase in proportion to the number of doctorally prepared nurses, very few have taken the responsibility to remedy this deficit by creating jobs which will motivate more nurses to seek doctoral education.

Many nurses in the past have not been particularly motivated to pursue doctoral education. Some nurses have attributed this situation to the lack of funds available for advanced education, while others have voiced their unwillingness to undertake advanced levels of education. Interesting, however, has been the charge by a group within the nursing profession that a major barrier has been the restricted nature of jobs available for the nurses with an earned doctoral degree. They point to the large number of doctorally prepared nurses who hold primarily academic or administrative positions and to the small number of this group who participate in clinical practice. It is true that nurses with doctoral degrees were traditionally isolated from clinical practice because of the desperate need for them in educational and administrative positions. The problem, however, is that this has become the established pattern for nurses with doctoral degrees and has perpetuated the detachment of these resources from the realities of clinical practice.

The question of the most effective utilization of doctorally prepared nurses is a challenge to service and education in nursing. Restriction of these nurses to primarily service or education perpetuates the artificial barriers which have been traditionally fostered in nursing and prevent the effective interface between the reality of practice and idealism of education. The exposure of nurses with earned doctoral degrees to nursing staff at all levels and to nursing students in the baccalaureate, master's and doctoral degree programs serves to prevent the isolation of nursing leaders from the pulsebeat of the profession.

Rush Medical Center is organized into a matrix structure designed to unify the academic and care elements into a holistic approach to health care delivery. The structure of the matrix is built to accord equality and parity among professionals in various disciplines. Beginning at the corporate level, this equity and parity is reflected throughout the organizational design and will be discussed in regard to the role of the nurse chairperson within the Rush Medical Center.

Purpose of Chairperson Role

The role of a doctorally prepared chairperson for each nursing department at Rush Medical Center evolved to bridge the artificial gap between practice and education. The role is based upon the underlying belief that clinical involvement is a prerequisite for health education and that the clinical area is a fertile resource for student learning and practice. Chairpersons are the recognized leaders for service and education within their departments and are expected to fully integrate patient care, education and research into the accomplishment of the goals of the department in conjunction with the goals of the Medical Center. Such a role is vital to the development of nursing at Rush and is considered an excellent springboard for future leadership roles such as deanships.

There is an underlying belief that clinical involvement is a prerequisite for health education and that the clinical area is a fertile resource for student learning and practice.

Actualization of Role

Actualization of the role of the nurse chairperson requires accountability for nursing and articulation of the department to the departments in the other colleges of the University and to other components of the Medical Center. At the chairperson level, there are built-in mechanisms to ensure integration between various disciplines, as well as a support system within the Division of Nursing which provides the chairperson with colleagues with whom to discuss complex issues and situations. The chairperson may be expected to solve complex management problems, initiate research projects and consult with the medical staff to resolve a critical issue which could impact the practice of nursing. A support system for the chairperson provides a source of strength and provides a resource for growth and the facilitation of change.

In the Division of Nursing the chairperson has several groups of support systems. As a chairperson of one of the seven specialty areas, the nurse has six other individuals with the same basic responsibility and accountability although the actual size of the department may vary. Each chairperson is a member of the Nursing Council which is the decision-making body of the Division of Nursing. This group includes leadership representatives from all areas in nursing and is regarded as a resource for consultation and decision making for nursing practice and education within the Rush Medical Center. There are additional opportunities for consultation and collaboration between chairpersons in nursing and their counterparts in the other colleges and other departments. Many chairpersons serve on University-wide committees and task forces and interface with each other in educational offerings and practice.

This wide range of activities provides the nurse chairperson with a diverse support system which promotes an atmosphere of colleagueship with individuals in similar roles. It also serves as a basis for negotiation and open communication between professionals whose primary goal is the provision of quality health care and education.

The role of the nurse chairperson at Rush Medical Center is not static because the individual is expected to make it work. Actualization of the role is dependent upon the nurse's ability to create an atmosphere that will be conducive to creative clinical practice and education. Total role expression for the nurse chairperson will result in the establishment of the role of the nurse as a unique contributor to excellence in health care delivery.

The professional power inherent in the role of the nurse chairperson at Rush is regarded as a positive force and an essential ingredient in effecting change. According to Claus and Bailey, power is "ability based on strength, willingness based on energy, and action that yields results."[1] These identified components of power are the basic ingredients of the total role expression of the nurse chairperson.

The strength of the role is derived from the ability of the individual nurse prepared at the doctoral level to utilize the full quantity of scientific knowledge and practice in both practice and educational realms of health care delivery. The willingness of the chairperson to implement the role is based upon the sincere commitment of the doctorally prepared nurse to increase nursing effectiveness through the full integration of practice, research, education and administration in cooperation with other health care providers. The action component of power for the nurse chairperson is the result of the integration and collaboration of nursing with other health professionals on a colleague level which in fact provides a shared power base.

The power of the nurse chairperson is a shared power model. Power for one chairperson empowers another and can result in a growth-producing atmosphere which increases professional effectiveness and strengthens the discipline of nursing.

On the wall of the psychiatric nursing department office hangs a poster which states. "We're all in this together." This may be one of the most subtle means we have of stating the department's philosophy, our way of operationalizing the Rush model of nursing. The chairperson is in a key position to facilitate excellence in nursing, as the role is pivotal in the matrix, both within nursing and for interdisciplinary negotiation. In a more traditional model, a department head might rely primarily on the head nurses for committee work, representing the department and so forth. In this matrix structure, the chairperson works through and with staff nurses, head nurses and assistants about equally, depending on the interest and needed expertise of a situation or problem.

Concurrently with their own clinical work, research, management and educational endeavors, chairpersons can perhaps best be described as the primary catalytic power people in each nursing department. By this concept we mean the power which ensues through the release of energy already in the system, e.g., helping to eliminate the hindrances to professional nurses carrying out the full spectrum of their role.[2] This might include such activities as finding budgetary support for continuing education activities, meeting with a staff nurse to discuss practice issues or negotiating with a peer in administration for improved support services (such as housekeeping).

Through the atmosphere of growth and the decentralized model, nurses establish relationships as professional colleagues rather than superiors-subordinates. Since all nurses in the department are operating within all four components of the professional role, separate "languages" and norms are not encouraged to develop and separate us. The resulting flow of communication enriches all levels. Of course, the communication can become more complex, leading to periods of frustration. As no role is free of frustration, however, it seems preferable to experience it in an atmosphere where helpless, one-down nursing has been replaced by interprofessional parity and collegiate support. We have found that viewing the role as a pioneer one, having faith in the operation of the matrix and maintaining a spirit of optimism are all powerful healers on a "lump-full" day. We have learned that when the model is not working, it is because we have reverted to working in premodel modes. Once this deficiency is corrected, we are on a smooth course again. Having been educated in more traditional models, we sometimes hesitate in operationalizing the behaviors needed in this role.

Skills Required

Our colleagues outside the Rush system have sometimes told us that the role of chairperson seems impossible, that it requires "supernurse" capabilities. We have been at it for a collective five years, and neither of us have developed an allergy to Kryptonite! We have identified, however, some behaviors that seem to facilitate implementation of the role of chairperson.

RISK TAKING

It seems apparent that if nurses are to grapple with the broad changes needed to bring us into the full professional arena, we need to begin to change old behavior patterns. This is the type of risk taking we refer to. Not chameleon-like changes in our personalities, but broader changes in style. Speaking out when we might have remained silent, acting rather than reacting, planning rather than drifting. We are attempting to develop in ourselves and in the department an atmosphere where questioning, discussing, and allowing latitude to handle one's own project from beginning to end are the norms. "Hover" supervision fosters dependence in the supervisee and stifles the supervisor. As a result of the growth of risk-taking behaviors, we have had some extremely creative problem solving. We have had a few creative failures, which has shown that there are no simple answers to complex problems. Yet the solution can fail while the experience itself is successful risk taking, increasing self-esteem for those who have swallowed hard and taken the leap. These experiences have led to the posting of the latest sign in the department office which reads: "To avoid criticism, do nothing, say nothing, BE NOTHING."

PRIORITY SETTING

Setting priorities is probably the most boring and overlooked section of any management text. Most of us are fairly sure we are able to do this quite well. The concept takes on new meaning, however, when one is consistently balancing the four components of the professional role. For example, which has the highest priority, attending an important nursing staff meeting on a unit or meeting with a faculty member (practitioner/teacher) regarding a problem with a student?

It is common for us to map out a week's, a month's, a year's and two or three year's priorities individually and in brainstorming sessions with the department. This gives direction to our activity. Once a plan is established, a necessary deviation is easier to manage.

SAYING "NO"

A common exercise in assertiveness training seminars is learning not to take on more jobs or responsibilities than one can manage concurrently. It is marvelous to help build a system that:

- fosters collegiate relationships so that others will take on tasks that we cannot do at one time or another;
- operates on the shared power model so different people taking on different tasks at different times is a positive aspect that supports the model;

- is dynamic and complex where opportunities consistently arise so that one absent is not felt as a loss.

Wisely managing time is an important component of the role of the chairperson.

CONCURRENCY

In transferring from the traditional management role to the chairperson role, we learned we needed new skills in being able to move quickly from one frame of reference to another. It is not usually possible to begin a task and work exclusively on that task to its end. One needs to be comfortable with several concurrent activities, many of which do not reach closure for a time. It is common to teach nursing students in the early morning, interview a staff nurse applicant, follow by functioning as a patient group therapist and perhaps attend a University committee meeting. This is not the concept sometimes referred to as "frequent hat switching," for in all these activities we are functioning from one role and one job, not parts of several jobs. As we move through the various activities, we are able to personally influence various elements of the system, as we are involved in all these elements. No more worry and helplessness about why doesn't "somebody" work to change a certain aspect of service or education. We are that somebody!

Positive Gains

One consistent problem in nursing management has been introducing change successfully.[3] An unanticipated (by us) outcome of the fusion of service and education has been a noticeable increase in the ability to effect change. Many of the issues addressed above have impact in this area. Another important factor has been that the composite picture obtained from being involved in both service and education and the input from peers in other disciplines of the matrix make us more sensitive to the timing of change. The appropriate timing of change may be the most important variable in eventual success. Not to be overlooked is the value of consistent involvement of all levels of nurses within the department. The collective professional knowledge of staff nurses, faculty and head nurses is phenomenal. High quality nursing care is the consistent result when this professional collective is focused through a common department, structure and endeavor.

An unanticipated outcome of the fusion of service and education has been a noticeable increase in the ability to effect change.

Decision making is experienced by the chairperson as both more simple and more complex than in a more traditional model. It is more simple in that decisions are made at the primary nurse and unit level rather than being sent up the chain and down again. Chairpersons may be called upon for input and expertise and are also expected to handle department-wide and matrix-level decisions. Decisions seem more complex at times because the concepts of shared power and matrix negotiation built into the system add numbers to the communication process. The chairperson needs skills in exercising the autonomy of the nursing role at Rush (no, no one else is going to negotiate or decide for you) and is responsible for encouraging the development of these skills in nurses throughout the department.

We are still discovering the positive gains of operationalizing this system. Some we have noted so far include a continuous stream of patients' and their families' letters and verbal praise of the care. Quality assurance measures have demonstrated many positive improvements in patient care. Also, in a recent survey of nursing staff, a majority of nurses cited high standards of patient care as a reason for their longevity at Rush.

The opportunity for exercise of the full professional role and professional parity has a geometric effect on nurses' enthusiasm, desire for continuing education and overall interest in professional growth. Nursing is taking its legitimate role in health care and its rightful place in the power hierarchy. The positive outcomes are seen throughout the matrix as nurses work collaboratively with other disciplines and are valued for their expertise.

A Vital Link

The doctorally prepared nurse chairperson serves as a vital link to bridge the artificial service–education gap. Skills of risk taking, setting careful priorities and managing time and resources have proven useful in putting this role into operation. The chairperson strives for excellence in all four components of the professional nursing role and in ensuring a milieu that encourages such excellence in the department. Rewards for this effort have been improved patient care, enthusiasm and professional growth of nursing staff and a legitimate share in the health care power hierarchy so that nurses value others and are valued for expertise in building better patient care.

"The power to animate all of life's seasons is a power that resides within (each of) us."[4]

REFERENCES

1. Claus, K. and Bailey, J. *Power and Influence in Health Care* (St. Louis: The C.V. Mosby Co. 1977) p. 3.
2. Munn, Y. "Power: How to Get It and Use It in Nursing today." *Nursing Administration Quarterly* 1:1 (Fall 1976) p. 95–103.
3. Leininger, M. "Political Nursing: Essential for Health Service and Educational Systems of Tomorrow." *Nursing Administration Quarterly* 2:3 (Spring 1978) p. 1–16.
4. Sheehy, G. *Passages* (New York: E.P. Dutton 1976) p. 354.

Ann Marie Brooks, R.N., D.N.Sc.
Chairperson
Psychiatric Nursing
Jane Ulsafer-Van Lanen, R.N., M.S.
Associate Chairperson
Psychiatric Nursing and Assistant Professor
Rush-Presbyterian-St. Luke's Medical Center
Chicago, Illinois

THE UNIT LEADER ROLE IN A MEDICAL INTENSIVE CARE UNIT

The unit leader role combines the concepts of education and service at the unit level. This position integrates the head nurse role with a faculty appointment. The unit leader role is an innovative approach intended to improve the quality of patient care.

This role provides leadership at the unit level on a daily basis through an individual with an increased knowledge base. The unit leader has the opportunity to analyze many influencing factors affecting unit function, utilizing the knowledge of graduate level preparation. This is in contrast to the usual role of the master's-prepared nurse in the clinical setting as an inservice coordinator or clinical specialist whose contact is intermittent or whose input tends to be assisting sporadically in dealing with specific problems or issues. The unit leader also has the opportunity to represent a highly clinical component of the nursing role within an educational setting. Thus the clinically-based individual can represent realistic concerns of nursing on educational, practice and research committees within the academic and hospital organizations. This individual offers a perspective influenced by graduate education and daily nursing experiences needed to meet the challenges and decisions such groups address. The involvement of the unit leader in the working unit and in the educational arena increases the opportunity for integration of the four components of the professional role, namely, service, education, consultation and research.

Functions of Unit Leader Role

The medical intensive care unit provides the ideal environment to develop and utilize the education-service role concept. Clinical expertise is required in dealing with the critically ill patient. A broad knowledge base is essential in maintaining clinical expertise in the highly technical and dynamic environment of the intensive care setting.

STAFF DEVELOPMENT

The intensive care setting frequently appeals to the young, often less experienced nurse. The highly technical environment will present a threatening situation to a new staff member. However, much emphasis is placed on the nurse's technical functioning by other professionals, patients and families. Patients and families gain a sense of comfort in observing a nurse who appears to be in control of the environment. Physicians emphasize the importance of knowing the "numbers," documenting the rhythm, producing the tracing and collecting specimens. Subjected to these diverse pressures, the nurse can easily become a sophisticated jack-of-all trades and master of none.

Initial emphasis must be focused on mastery of required skills to function optimally in this environment. New staff members generally identify only these technical aspects as a learning need. With organized, directed assistance these technical functions can be readily mastered, and the nurse can practice these skills appropriately and competently. Skill mastery alone, however, does not produce a professional nurse.

As unit leader one must assist the staff in developing a professional aspect of the nursing role. Identification of scientific theory required to utilize the information collected and provision of opportunities to meet these educational needs becomes a major focus of the unit leader. By broadening the knowledge base of the staff nurse, a more sophisticated level of nursing practice can be identified by patients and other professionals in the setting.

In order to develop this theoretical base, many concepts must be introduced to, and reinforced in, the staff. The educational focus could easily maintain an emphasis on medical and physiological principles and concepts. However, to develop a more sophisticated level of nursing practice, the nurse must incorporate concepts and ideas from other schools in planning and implementing care. Theories related to crisis, pain, sleep, environment, communication, behavior modification, adult or child learning, teaching and many others should be utilized in nursing practice.

To develop a more sophisticated level of nursing practice, the nurse must incorporate concepts and ideas from other schools in planning and implementing care.

A typical example of the need for the integration of skill and knowledge involves the patient presenting with cardiogenic shock requiring hemodynamic monitoring and intra-aortic balloon pumping. Initially, technical skills and collection of physiological data are vital in stabilization of the patient. The stress of the ICU environment, threat of death, separation from significant others, continual disturbances depriving the patient of rest, decreased nutritional intake, recurrence of pain, territorial invasion by strangers and loss of control over the situation are all factors that must also be addressed by the primary nurse. Data collection routines can be altered in order to meet the needs of the patient while maintaining adequate surveillance. Medications can be scheduled to correspond with other required treatments in order to decrease the frequency of disturbances. Treatments and procedures should be scheduled with consideration of visiting hours, meals or rest periods. Consideration of these factors will improve the quality of patient care and the level of nursing practice.

BEHAVIOR MODELING

The unit leader assists the staff in developing a broader knowledge base by presenting as a strong behavior model, providing opportunities for learning, evaluating staff performance regularly and providing constructive reinforcement frequently. Through the integration of technical skills and knowledge the staff will learn to demonstrate nursing practice as professional nurses, not as technically competent data collectors.

DEFINING THE NURSING ROLE

The ICU setting offers many distractions in which the nursing focus can be lost. Another aspect of a unit leader's role is to assist with defining the nursing role in this setting. As medical care and therapeutic interventions become more specialized and complex, many more providers are entering the health care settings. Issues frequently arise concerning identification of the group to perform a certain function. Consideration must be given to who is qualified and available who will also accept accountability and responsibility for performing the function in question. Other professionals within the hospital are often strong forces in assigning these functions to nursing. The presenting argument usually involves the 24-hour-a-day availability of nurses, the ease in teaching them, and their established responsibility for the patients. However, close examination must be made of the function in question and its relationship to nursing practice. The unit leader does not have to be eager to accept additional tasks to prove the capabilities of nursing. With a more developed concept of nursing practice based on education and clinical expertise, the unit leader can assist in identifying the nursing role to other professionals and can also assist staff nurses in defining their roles in interactions with other members of the health team.

The following was recently an issue in our medical intensive care unit. When hemodynamic monitoring was an infrequent diagnostic intervention, nurses accepted the responsibility of equipment preparation and care. As the sophistication of the unit developed, however, the volume and variety of machinery began to increase and the time required for machine care also greatly increased. It quickly became clear to nursing leadership that what was once a rare and short-term event was becoming a standard operating procedure and required excessive nursing time for nonnursing functions. Negotiations were begun with the monitoring personnel initially to develop justification for developing a technician role, later to identify job descriptions and currently to clarify nursing and technician functions and areas of overlap. Although we have developed and implemented the technician role, there still exist areas of debate and need for further clarification. We have, however, addressed the major issue, nursing identification of its role in this question.

MODELING BEHAVIOR

A major function of the unit leader is to present a behavioral model for the nursing staff and students. Incorporation of technical and conceptual aspects of nursing care becomes easier to identify when observed in practice. The unit leader appreciates the frustrations of the staff nurse when functioning at the bedside. Staff and students also have the opportunity to observe the unit leader deal with the frustrations they experience. In some situations, consultants may be utilized to deal with particular problems. The unit leader should be aware of available resources and utilize them. The staff and students not only become aware of the resources available but also how to incorporate the consultants' role into their practice. By observing the unit leader identify a need for assistance in dealing with problems, it becomes easier for the staff to recognize and acknowledge their needs for assistance.

The unit leader also has a responsibility to present a behavioral model as a leader and decision maker. Many issues can be shared with the staff and alternatives discussed. Both short- and long-term effects of the alternatives should be identified in the discussions. Leadership skills must be practiced and developed as any other skill is developed. Once again the unit leader assists staff and student development of the professional nursing role by providing knowledge and the opportunity to practice leadership skills. The unit leader always retains ultimate responsibility and accountability for decisions and results. However, delegation of tasks and responsibilities with supervision and direction develops leadership and decision-making skills. As the individual's skills develop, projects or duties delegated become more complex. Eventually various staff members will build skill and confidence in both decision-making and leadership functions, thereby increasing the strength and functioning capabilities within the unit. Various projects can be undertaken simultaneously through utilization of the delegation process.

Currently various staff nurses on our unit are coordinating several projects, including the writing of an orientation guide for new staff, a hemodynamic manual of policies and procedures and the development of guidelines for peer review among the staff. These projects give staff the opportunity to develop leadership and administrative skills. Their involvement in these projects also has generated an increased commitment to nursing practice.

ESTABLISHING UNIT ATMOSPHERE AND PACE

The unit leader has the responsibility of establishing the atmosphere and pace of the unit. By increasing the staff's knowledge and skills, higher standards can be established. In turn, these standards become reflected in a more sophisticated level of nursing practice. The overall effect is a stronger sense of professionalism and identity as a nurse and an increase in quality of care. As an entire unit develops this sense of identity, commitment and pride are generated by the level of practice performed within the unit. This reinforces the higher level of practice.

The Unit Leader—A Challenging Role

The integration of the unit leader role into an agency can be challenging. A unit leader's role involves considerable change which frequently results in stress on the change agent as well as on the system being changed.

Frequently, identification of role functions and boundaries for the unit leader are unclear and must be developed and established.

The role itself is still developing. Frequently, identification of role functions and boundaries are unclear and must be developed and established. It is also a very time-consuming position requiring considerable commitment and involvement. However imperfect this system may seem, its disadvantages are far overshadowed by the advantages. The amount of accomplishment sensed as the role is implemented, and the level of nursing practice that is developed, cannot be realized in any other system. The potential for development of professional power within this framework seems both apparent and necessary to ensure quality nursing care.

Roberta Fruth, R.N., M.S.
Unit Leader
Department of Medical Nursing
Rush-Presbyterian-St. Luke's Medical Center
Chicago, Illinois

The Adjunct Appointment Can Provide Realistic Experience for Leadership Students

Claire Meisenheimer, R.N., M.S.N.
Assistant Vice President
Quality Assurance
Froedtert Memorial Lutheran Hospital
Milwaukee, Wisconsin
Former Director
Education Department
Family Hospital
Adjunct Clinical Assistant Professor
University of Wisconsin-Milwaukee
Milwaukee, Wisconsin

NURSING EDUCATORS versus nursing administrators, professionals versus technicians, quality patient care, cost effectiveness, dearth of leadership—these issues of concern fill the nursing literature. A significant way to address these concerns is through the use of adjunct appointments to teach nursing leadership.

The concept of adjunct or shared positions is not new, nor is the fact that professional nurses have always assumed leadership and managerial responsibilities in providing quality patient care. But incorporating these aspects of nursing into nursing curricula and ensuring that nursing education programs provide both theory and practice in the management-leadership function remains a largely unrealized task.

BACKGROUND INFORMATION AND THEORY

The complexity of contemporary medicine and of hospital structures has produced the convergence at the patient's bedside of numerous specialized individuals to provide patient care. All of these individuals, relating directly or indirectly to the patient, perform a function—be it diagnostic, therapeutic, supportive or other—and leave. The nurse is the only one who is really responsible for and can manage the coordination and continuity of patient care. Distinguishing between the nurse's own independent patient care function and the management of others directly and indirectly providing care is frequently a source of a role conflict for the new nurse manager.

The nurse manager function is an important one. Like every other role within the hospital, it is a product of processes and relationships which permeate the entire organization. Therefore, new graduates must perceive their role as nurse managers not in isolation, but as part of an interaction process involving organizational function, occupational specialization and a complex of formal and informal role behavior. However, today's nursing education is not providing adequate preparation for the nurse's management role. Programs emphasize learning how to provide good patient care, but give little attention to developing skills necessary to influence organizational goals and design.[1] Nurses are not provided with concepts of management and nursing theory that prepare them to plan, organize, implement and evaluate ongoing activities related to patient care. Present curricula are developed around a core of knowledge and the nurse's independent care function. After graduation, however, nurses cannot function alone and independently, but must develop the ability to coordinate their own work with that of other nursing personnel and other workers within the health care system.

With an understanding of the hospital's bureaucratic organization and processes, the skills and abilities necessary for nurses to function as first-level managers can be identified.

There has been and continues to be a great dichotomy between the bureaucratic hospital organization and the professional person who performs within such an organization. Graves, using the term "bureaucratic" to describe a particular way of organizing human activity, says that "a bureaucracy is a system with a hierarchical structure of authority, a clear-cut division of labor, and a formal system of rules and regulations to govern official decisions and actions."[2]

Nurses need to recognize and understand the necessary aspects of bureaucratic structuring and regulations; at the same time, they must be adequately prepared to combat excessive and unnecessarily confining bureaucratic pressures. Nurses need to have input into this bureaucratic organization by planning programs and systems which define the nature and intent of nursing care practices.[3] But students who are educated to care for patients without formal responsibility for their actions and without formal

Nursing students who are educated to care for patients without formal responsibility for their actions and without formal commitment by the organization to their role become graduates who have little sense of their own personal authority.

commitment by the organization to their role become the graduates who have little sense of their own personal authority.

Identifying Management

Management—the people involved and the procedures followed—has been identified as the main factor influencing the success or failure of organizations. The study of management in nursing education often focuses on leadership rather than on general management theories. Leadership, administration and management are not identical. Distinguishing between administration and management, Alexander states that administration "is responsible for the determination of the aims for which an organization and its management are to strive, which establishes the broad policies under which they are to operate, and which gives general oversight to the continuing effectiveness of the total operation in reaching the objectives sought."[4]

Management is the process and agency which directs and guides an organization's operation in the realizing of established aims.[5]

Management, as defined by Terry, "is a distinct process consisting of planning, organizing, actuating, controlling, performed to determine and accomplish stated objectives by the use of human beings and other resources."[6] Management, using this definition, denotes an activity; those who perform this activity are managers. Nurse managers then are managers because they are accountable for the planning and coordination of all persons who relate directly or indirectly to the patient.

Leading human beings is an important part of actuating efforts. Terry defines leadership as a "complex relationship existing between the leader, the led, the organization, and the social values and economic and political conditions."[7] The ability to influence others derives from the relationships and interactions the leader can effect. The term leadership is sometimes used as if it were an attribute of personality, sometimes as if it were a characteristic of certain positions and sometimes as an attribute of behavior. There seem to be distinct conceptual advantages to defining leadership in behavioral terms as an act of influence on a matter of organization relevance.[8] June Bailey and her associates at the University of California, San Francisco, have developed an operational definition of leadership:

> . . . as a set of actions that influence members of a group to move toward goal setting and goal attainment. Inherent in the actions are situational variables; personal, organizational, and social power bases; formal and func-

tional bases of authority; and accountability. Other elements in the spectrum of leadership actions are sound managerial and human relations behaviors and the use of influence strategies that will promote a willingness to follow so that individual and organizational goals can be achieved. Thus, leadership is viewed as multidimensional, encompassing the wise use of power, managerial functions, and human relations processes.[9]

Identifying Leadership

Leadership, accordingly, can only be defined by the behaviors manifested by leaders or by role enactment, and not by leadership characteristics. However, Terry states that such factors as the "leader's personality, skill, experience, confidence, awareness of self, type of followers, interactions, and organization climate influence the leader's behavior and what he does or does not accomplish."[10]

Certain words and phrases often are associated with leadership: organizational effectiveness, goal-oriented behavior, decision making, creative risk taking, change "agentry," political strategy and systems analysis. These phrases certainly are not the ones usually associated with caring: empathy, comfort measures, mother-surrogate role, socializing agent and emotional support.[11] The education structure for nurses is usually caring oriented with little emphasis on the total perspective of management. In order to function in the real world, today's nurse needs an understanding of both sets of characteristics.

Finally, it should be pointed out that at present most nursing educators are somewhat removed from reality. They frequently teach an idealized version of the work setting. Armstrong states that "many new graduates begin work with a wealth of knowledge but limited clinical experience; they are more educationally oriented than service oriented to the role and responsibilities they are expected to assume."[12] Therein lies the professional-bureaucratic conflict. It is essential that nursing education develop both clinical expertise and strategies for implementing clinical programs.

They must also be able to identify their autonomous professional role—and be provided with the opportunity to experience this role prior to graduation—in order to provide for, and assist others in providing for, the core professional function: managing patient care.

THE UNIVERSITY OF WISCONSIN-MILWAUKEE CURRICULUM

At University of Wisconsin-Milwaukee (UWM), we have developed and incorporated into the nursing education curriculum a course designed to teach administrative, management and leadership skills. Introduction to Nursing Leadership, a six-credit course, is taught to senior nursing students. It seeks to provide a milieu in which students can be creative, develop independence and prepare themselves for the real work world.

The course is divided into theory (lecture two hours per week), group discussions (one hour per week), clinical experiences (six hours per week), and independent study and a leadership analysis paper. Credit allocation is as follows:

Theory
Independent study—one credit
Leadership analysis and midterm exam—one credit
Final exam—one credit

Practice
Clinical—two credits
Discussion—one credit

The stated goal of the course is to provide the student with an opportunity to:

1. observe, analyze and participate in various aspects of leadership as it relates to management, delivery and evaluation of nursing; and
2. develop skills in an independent study.[13]

Orientation

Systematic orientation of students to the clinical agency is quite lengthy. The students must be exposed to a great deal of information and many persons. These include administrative persons within the agency—i.e., the executive director, the director of nursing, the administrator of finance and department heads—and various persons in support systems. Persons in line and staff positions discuss their unique roles and relationships. How the staff nurse interfaces with each discipline and each department in providing patient care is basic to these discussions.

Organizational structure, roles and relationships, power and authority, communication systems, financial accountability, and models of decision making and change are examined during orientation and throughout the semester. The practical applications of research are discussed in the hope of stimulating students to make research part of their independent study.

The first 30 hours of the clinical experience are on the structured "orientation" basis, thus lessening the students' anxiety. Approximately 70 hours are left for the students to plan independently. Depending upon area of interest, they may choose experiences within or outside the agency. They must write objectives for what they choose and evaluate their experiences based upon those objectives. As the semester progresses, the students' increased ability for more accurate self-assessment also reflects their independent judgment and leadership skills.

Flexibility

There is flexibility as to how the course objectives can be met. Group discussions have been utilized in several courses. The students felt a need one spring semester for a different group experience and chose to provide a workshop for other nursing students instead. The topic was stress and relaxation. Group process was facilitated by all the students accepting responsibility for a portion of the workshop. The professor attended only the initial meeting and the dress rehearsal; two students were designated as responsible for keeping her informed. The workshop was evaluated by the students. All received the same grade, a policy determined at the outset.

Independent projects are usually valued at one credit, but may be negotiated with the instructor for two credits. If the project is of this magnitude, the student's clinical time may be reduced by half. Students are encouraged to plan, organize, implement and evaluate a project which is meaningful to them as well as the agency. Patient education materials, teaching models, quality assurance programs and other such projects are usually used by the agency for future programming. Thus both the student and the agency benefit.

Students are really increasing their self-awareness at this point. Philosophies are discussed in depth, and personal philosophies are written down and contrasted with those of the organization and of society. Self-awareness and congruency of organizational and employee values are emphasized. Students are sufficiently oriented to bureaucratic beliefs to be able to function effectively within an organization and create change.

As students begin to integrate these new concepts, an appreciation for the consumer of health emerges. In becoming a member of the health care team, public control and accountability become very real issues. Students learn that professional nurses must collaboratively plan to provide and evaluate care with the patient and other appropriate members of the team. They examine the health care system and their leadership role within it.

Nursing students need experiences that will provide for their greatest growth, experiences as close as possible to the real situations in which they will work after graduation. Until nursing provides practitioners with apprenticeships similar to those in other professions, the adjunct appointment can help fill the education-service gap.

Nursing students need experiences that will provide for their greatest growth, experiences as close as possible to the real situations in which they will work after graduation.

COLLABORATION (See Figure 1)

In 1929 Annie W. Goodrich affiliated the Yale School of Nursing with the New Haven Hospital. Faculty functioned in every hospital department where students were assigned.

FIGURE 1. SERVICE-EDUCATION COLLABORATION

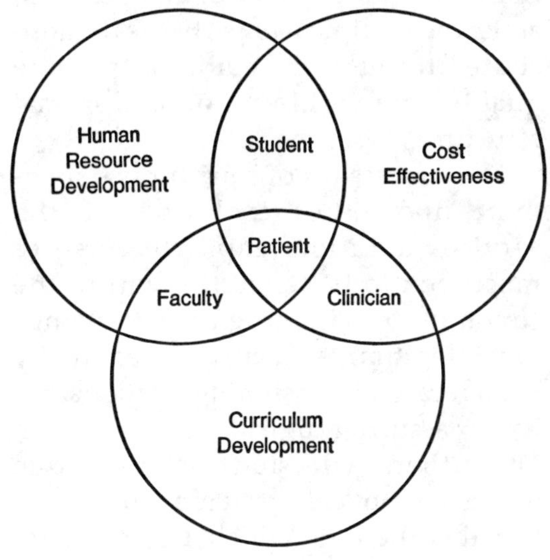

The educational director of the New Haven Visiting Nurses' Association was also a member of the faculty.[14] The University of Florida patterned its program after the medical organizational model in the early 1960s.[15]

In August 1966 the Department of Nursing of University Hospitals of Cleveland, and the Frances Payne Bolton School of Nursing of Case Western Reserve University embarked on a five-year experiment partially funded by the W. K. Kellogg Foundation.[16-20] They defined "three types of joint appointments—leadership-clinical, faculty associate, and shared salary—each one determined by the responsibilities held by the appointee in relation to the school and the hospital."[21]

The University of Rochester in 1971 integrated the School of Nursing and the Nursing Service Department under the leadership of the dean of nursing. Powers states that the joint appointee position within the unification model "has been most evident in the development of a profession, rather than a bureaucratic organization.[22]

The appointment presently held by the author at the UWM is similar to the leadership-clinical appointment at Case Western Reserve University. Family Hospital, the primary appointment (60 percent), receives salary reimbursement from UWM (40 percent)—thus paying salary and all fringe benefits.

BENEFITS OF THE JOINT APPOINTEE

The joint appointee is committed to the profession of nursing: practice, education and research. The understanding of organizational structure—informal, as well as formal—promotes administrative support in developing this new role. Knowledge and experience in teaching, as well as clinical competency, is necessary.

There must be participation in curriculum development, and appropriate committees in both settings in order to effectively create change. Credibility is demonstrated when students are able to apply theory to their practice.

If nurses are really to be managers of patient care, then universities must provide students the opportunities to examine the management process. The author's role as a resource person, consultant and facilitator allows the student freedom to be creative within a supportive system. Until this point in time, the students rarely practice without constant supervision. They are now able to spend longer periods of time on nursing units, working more closely with staff nurses, families and other members of the health care team, and to observe and frequently participate on committees. They can apply change and decision-making models to practice.

Joint appointments are a cost-effective mechanism for both agencies when salaries are shared for time and expertise. The university can provide appropriate faculty for staff development and continuing education programs, patient education materials (hardware and software) and research assistance. Clinical expertise is demonstrated through the ability to provide quality care within an organizational structure.

The profession of nursing is dependent upon the resolution of the service-education gap. Universities must look to the expertise within the community, while the service agency must legitimize faculty expertise by collaboratively assuming responsibility for assuring high standards of care. Only then will students have role models who can provide an educational milieu in which the management of patients can be practiced.

REFERENCES

1. McBride, A. et al. "Leadership in Nursing: Problems and Possibilities in Nursing." *American Journal of Nursing* 72:8 (August 1972) p. 1445.
2. Graves, H. H. "Can Nursing Shed Bureaucracy?" *American Journal of Nursing* 71:3 (March 1971) p. 491.
3. Erickson, E. H. "Are Nurses Needed for Administration or Management in Hospitals?" *Journal of Nursing Administration* 4:4 (July–August 1974) p. 21.
4. Alexander, E. L. *Nursing Administration in the Hospital Health Care System* (St. Louis: The C.V. Mosby Co. 1971) p. 91.
5. Ibid.
6. Terry, G. R. *Principles of Management* (Homewood, Ill.: Richard D. Irwin, Inc. 1972) p. 4.
7. Ibid. p. 461.
8. Christman, L. B. "Nursing Leadership—Style and Substance." *American Journal of Nursing* 67:10 (October 1967) p. 2091.
9. Claus, K. E. and Bailey, J. T. *Power and Influence in Health Care: A New Approach to Leadership* (St. Louis: The C.V. Mosby Co. 1977) p. 5.
10. Terry. *Principles of Management* p. 464.
11. McBride et al. *"Leadership in Nursing: Problems and Possibilities in Nursing"* p. 1445.
12. Armstrong, M. L. "Bridging the Gap Between Graduation and Employment." *Journal of Nursing Administration* 4:6 (November–December 1974) p. 42.
13. Course Syllabus, University of Wisconsin-Milwaukee, 1977–1978.
14. Powers, M. J. "The Unification Model in Nursing." *Nursing Outlook* 24:8 (August 1976) p. 482–487.
15. Smith, D. M. "Education and Service Under Our Administration." *Nursing Outlook* 13:2 (February 1965) p. 54–56.
16. Pierik, M. M. "Experiment to Effect Change," *Supervisor Nurse* 2:4 (April 1971) p. 69–75.
17. Pierik, M. M. "Joint Appointments: Collaboration for Better Patient Care." *Nursing Outlook* 21:9 (September 1973) p. 576–579.
18. Schlotfeldt, R. M. and MacPhail, J. "An Experiment in Nursing: Rationale and Characteristics." *American Journal of Nursing* 69:5 (May 1969) p.

1018–1023.

19. Schlotfeldt, R. M. and MacPhail, J. "An Experiment in Nursing: Introducing Planned Change." *American Journal of Nursing* 69:6 (June 1969) p. 1247–1252.
20. Schlotfeldt, R. M. and MacPhail, J. "Experiment in Nursing: Implementing Planned Change." *American Journal of Nursing* 69:7 (July 1969) p. 1475–1480.
21. Pierik. "Joint Appointments: Collaboration for Better Patient Care."
22. Powers. "The Unification Model in Nursing."

SUGGESTED READINGS

MacPhail, J. "Promoting Collaboration Between Education and Service." *The Canadian Nurse* 71:5 (May 1975) p. 32–34.

Walker, V. and Hawkins, J. "Management: A Factor in Clinical Nursing." *Nursing Outlook* 13:2 (February 1965) p. 57–58.

Pitfalls in Developing Nurse Internship Programs

Joan Gygax Spicer, R.N., M.S.N.
Consultant
Spicer and Spicer Associates
San Jose, California

IN THE SERVICE sphere of nursing we are still debating the relative clinical adeptness of nurses prepared at diploma- versus associate-degree versus baccalaureate-degree levels. While the emotional debate continues, the immediate circumstances need attention: a discrepancy exists between the clinical competencies possessed by graduate nurses and the clinical competencies required of them by employers.

This discrepancy is referred to as the education–service split. As a result, support programs must be provided to help graduate nurses acquire the repertoire of skills they need to function in the hospital setting. These programs are being called by such names as Nurse Internship, R.N. I., Preceptorship and Individualized Orientation. In contrast to hospital orientation programs—which are designed to enable nurses to function within particular institutions—nurse internships are aimed at assisting nurses to function within the *profession.* (Although the rudiments of these programs predate Kramer,[1] their scientific basis is her research on the transition from graduate nurse to staff nurse.)

Nurse internship programs financially supported by the service organization are a new area for nursing and present pitfalls for nursing administrators. The demands on their time are great, and it is difficult for them to be totally on top of every issue. Certain potentially difficult aspects of developing nurse internship programs should be given careful consideration.

PROGRAM OUTCOMES: POSITIVE AND NEGATIVE CONSIDERATIONS

Several factors make investment in nurse internship programs potentially worthwhile:

- Nurse internship programs enhance the spontaneous nursing adeptness in assessment and intervention that is demanded by the trend toward increased acuity of the hospitalized patient population.
- Nurse internships serve to compensate for the prevailing education–service split.
- Nurse internships may reduce turnover among graduate nurses (identified as contributing greatly to the documented staff nurse turnover rate of 70 percent nationwide).[2]
- Nurse internships may be useful in recruitment.

Giving only cursory consideration to these factors is dangerous because it leaves possible negative ramifications inadequately defined.

The Education–Service Split

Once the decision is made to develop a nurse internship program, delegating the project to the nursing education (nursing inservice) department is the natural next step. The nursing education department provides an important check in the checks and balances of the nursing division and therefore requires a degree of autonomy. It is from the work of this department that a standard knowledge base is maintained from which all nurses in the institution function. However, unless nursing administrators hold the nursing education department accountable for responding to service needs, they risk recreating the education–service split at the institutional level, and the nurse internship program may fall victim to it. Because concern about the educa-

Unless nursing administrators hold the nursing education department accountable for responding to service needs, they risk creating an education-service split and the nursing internship program may fall victim to it.

tion–service relationship has been focused so long at the community level, there is a real danger of ignoring a possible split at the institutional level.

Turnover

Turnover is affected by controllable and uncontrollable variables. A nurse internship program is not necessarily the proper remedy. Reasons for turnover have to be explored beyond what is stated on termination papers. Are nurses leaving because of marriage, pregnancy or relocation? Or is the turnover related to factors such as desire to pursue formal education, lack of professional growth, poor interpersonal professional relationships or inadequate nurse managers? Are nurses relocating or just working in other nearby hospitals as an escape? If professional growth opportunities are provided in work settings or if work settings are made flexible to facilitate the nurses' formal education efforts, will nurses still disengage completely from the work settings to pursue formal education? Are nurse manager actions that contribute to turnover even identified and dealt with? The direct supervisors of staff nurses are the most crucial level in the nursing administrative structure and usually the least prepared to manage professional employees. Nurse internship programs address only the turnover related to the difficulties of adjustment of the graduate nurse during the transition to staff nurse; to expect more is to invite disappointment.

Recruitment

Marketing internship programs for recruitment attracts the shoppers in an employees' market and enlarges the selection pool of nurses in the employers' market. Overemphasis on recruitment or misplaced emphasis on the recruiting process sometimes leads to: financial difficulties in program operations because funds are shifted from program operations to the recruitment program; insufficient attention to nurses presently in the program in favor of potential candidates; possible deception of the nursing administrator and nurses entering the program by letting actual program objectives get lost in the marketing process.

FACTORS IN INTERNSHIP PROGRAM SUCCESS

Regular Staff as a Primary Resource

Program objectives can be attained only if adequate resources are available. The most vital resource is nursing personnel, particularly the person who will serve as program coordinator. Pitfalls can be avoided if the coordinator is mature and adequately versed in the coordinator role. But lack of understanding often causes the coordinator to reinforce a teacher-student relationship that fosters dependence, instead of encouraging and establishing a nurse–facilitator relationship that promotes independence. The coordinator's teacher role may influence program candidate selection toward nurses who want a dependent student role instead of an independent staff nurse role.

In the nurse–facilitator relationship the coordinator's primary aim is to foster the development of strong bonds: (1) among staff nurses and (2) between staff nurses and head nurses. Although initially the nurse intern identifies with the coordinator, this relationship has to be replaced by the other bonds before the program is completed.

Nonintern staff nurses have to be included in the focus of the program; otherwise its objectives will be defeated. Existing staff members must see the need for the program and have input into it. Program content should be made available to them before it is used with the new nurses; an opportune time to do this is during inservice sessions. If regular staff are not made familiar with the program, anxiety over the unknown arises and can be negatively channeled. In addition, if all the attention is given to the new nurses, the equivalent of sibling jealousy is created in the more senior nurses.

Nonintern staff nurses have to be included in the focus of the internship program; otherwise its objectives will be defeated.

Program Content and Format

A common pitfall in designing nurse internship programs is to select content and materials that are part of *basic* nursing programs. Nursing administrators must hold new nurses accountable for basic nursing knowledge—to preserve the new nurses' self-images as well as to avoid becoming financially responsible for providing a review of the basic nursing program. The internship program design has to allow the nurses to work with their existing knowledge base in managing assignments, setting priorities and intervening in changing clinical status situations. Since it is difficult to add to an inactive knowledge base, what the nurses have already learned must first be activated; then more information may be provided. Program content should include "cookbook" information. To assist nurses through the time when they are still activating their knowledge base, they need drilling in rote memory of the phases in a patient's change in clinical status: what is happening, the signs and symptoms presented and nursing responsibilities in intervention.[3]

To promote the new nurses' independence and to foster staff relationships, the program structure should minimize the amount of time nurse interns are required to be away from the patient care unit. The use of preceptors working in a one-to-one ratio with new nurses on the patient care unit for a large portion of the program should be considered. Using preceptors benefits not only new nurses but also existing staff by helping to develop staff relationships. The use of preceptors also promotes what

Erikson refers to as "generativity" within the nursing profession.[4]

AVOIDING THE PITFALLS

Existing weaknesses in the nursing system have to be identified to prevent the nurse internship program from becoming the "whipping boy" or from being misconstrued as the cause of the problems. The nursing administrator should plan on using extra time and energy to attend to internal problems which are likely to be exposed on the patient care units during the process of the program.

Nursing administrators who decide to implement nurse internship programs have many obscure factors to consider to avoid pitfalls. They also make a symbolic commitment to support change—in that nurse internship programs are change processes and their ultimate outcome is not only change in nursing, but change touching all disciplines in the hospital.

REFERENCES

1. Kramer, M. *Reality Shock: Why Nurses Leave Nursing* (Saint Louis: The C.V. Mosby Co. 1974).
2. National Commission on Nursing and Nursing Education. *An Abstract for Action* (New York: McGraw-Hill Book Co. 1970) p. 132-137.
3. Spicer, J. G. "Help for the Staff Nurse in Crisis." *Supervisor Nurse* 9:9 (September 1978) p. 82-83.
4. Erikson, E. *Identity and the Life Cycle: Psychological Issues* (New York: International Universities Press 1959).

Perspectives on Nursing Education: The Transition Process

COLLABORATION IS THE KEY ELEMENT

"BEING A NURSE is not quite the same as becoming one!"[1] How does one transcend the awesome period between student and professional nurse? Does the educational institution provide relevant learning experiences for nursing students to become autonomous practitioners? Does the service agency provide a supportive climate for nurses to become lifelong learners? And are nurses committed to the development and modification of theory to practical implementation? If education and service are working toward the same goal—the development of an individual who can provide quality patient care—why does this chasm exist?

Nurse educators and nurse administrators have long recognized and discussed the difficulties with which new graduate nurses assume their first professional position. The dilemma in nursing can be identified as the issue of whose responsibility it is to ascertain what the beginning practitioner's clinical competency should be in meeting the needs of patients.

Nursing education and service each represent a horn of the dilemma, for both educators and administrators feel their special knowledge and experience give them a prerogative. If we want to resolve the dilemma, communication must exist.

Education and service must collaborate and stop being hypercritical of each other's policies and practices. (See Figure 1.) Educators, whose primary goal is to provide relevant learning experiences for nursing students, must be sensitive to the common goal of nursing in providing quality patient care. Service agencies need to provide a support climate in which students can be allowed flexibility and many opportunities for independent decision making. Education and service must no longer be guests in each other's houses. They must commit themselves to common goals and learn to trust and respect each other by promoting increased interaction.

Education and service must commit themselves to common goals and learn to trust and respect each other by promoting increased interaction.

FIGURE 1. THE ART OF COLLABORATION

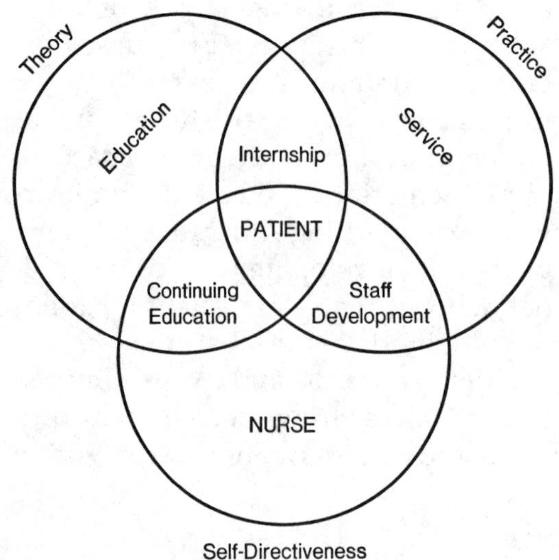

An educator, who is committed to maintaining clinical competence and assuming responsibility for providing quality patient care submits the following mechanisms for resolving our dilemma. (See "Easing The Transition From Classroom into Clinical Setting—Implications for Education," this article.)

Service agencies that employ new graduates must accept the responsibility for developing young nurses as professional practitioners while at the same time providing continuous quality nursing care to the patient. Service agencies must recognize that no school or type of nursing education program can possibly prepare nurses for all hospital situations.[2] They need to be aware that differences do exist between types of programs, between programs themselves, between clinical facilities and of course between individuals. Representatives from the associate degree, diploma and baccalaureate programs cannot be considered equal either in their educational preparation for practice or in their ability to perform effectively in the service setting.

However, research has shown that no distinction is made. Frequently, orientation, supervision, work assignments and charge experiences are the same for all nurses. Service must provide a broader scope than just orientation to the facility, equipment and routines; more than working with another staff member; more than periodic meetings on special procedures. There must be methods for facilitating this transition to graduate nurse status and the integration of new graduates into the "real" work situation.

One alternative that has been implemented at Family Hospital is the Nurse Internship Program. (See "Easing the Transition from Classroom into Clinical Setting—Implications for Service," this article.)

The support and guidance new graduates have experienced in the internship should emphasize and internalize their responsibility for continued learning. The publication of various standards for fulfilling the profession's responsibilities in providing quality care is placing a greater value on competency. Administration is recognizing and supporting educational designs based on the learning needs of nursing staff. Philosophies congruent with employees and the organization have been developed. The organizational structure identifies the education department function and provides for accountability through role descriptions of appropriate personnel.

Cost accountability is a major issue in the health care system today. Value placed on staff development and continuing education is demonstrated with adequate budgeting for competent staff and physical resources. Provisions must be made for financial and time compensations with expectations and responsibilities clearly defined.

It is increasingly apparent that the time has come for nursing education and service to narrow the existing gap. Both must assume responsibility for guaranteeing quality standards of care in health settings used for student practice.

The development of joint appointments would enhance relationships and promote increased interaction between representatives of two or more organizations. Shared responsibility for the quality of care rendered would necessitate definition of roles and relationships with the position being viewed as one job. Participation in meetings, serving on committees and contributing to curriculum development would provide both types of specialists mechanisms for influencing standards of practice. Appropriate utilization of these role models should provide the opportunity for continued learning of students, staff and patients.

Collaboration must occur for the good of the patient, the good of the practitioner and the good of the profession.

REFERENCES

1. Peplau, H. E. "An Open Letter to a New Graduate." *Nursing Digest* 3:2 (March–April 1975) p. 36.
2. Lambertson, E. "No School Can Prepare Nurses For All the Hospital Situations." *Modern Hospital* 112:2 (February 1969) p. 127.

SUGGESTED READINGS

Brock, M. "Bridging the Gap Between Service and Education." *Supervisor Nurse* 5:7 (July 1974) p. 27–34.

Murphy, J. S. "The Dilemma in Nursing Practice." *Journal of Nursing Administration* 4:1 (January–February 1974) p. 16–18.

Rosendahl, P. "Self-Direction For Learners: An Andragogical Approach to Nursing Education." *Nursing Forum* 13:2 (1974).

Tobin, H. M. *The Process of Staff Development: Components for Change* (St. Louis: The C.V. Mosby Co. 1974).

Vogelberger, M. "The Professional Adjustment and Growth of the New Graduate." *The Journal of Continuing Education in Nursing* 2:5 (September–October 1971) p. 21–27.

Claire Meisenheimer, R.N., M.S.N.
Assistant Vice President, Quality Assurance
Froedtert Memorial Lutheran Hospital
Milwaukee, Wisconsin

EASING THE TRANSITION FROM CLASSROOM INTO CLINICAL SETTING—IMPLICATIONS FOR EDUCATION

The effectiveness of an educational program must be judged by things that happen after the students graduate.

The present dilemma in nursing education seems to be one of teaching all there is to know about nursing—and more—in a period of four years or less. It is small wonder that the graduates of our nation's nursing programs enter their first job situation as professionals feeling overwhelmed and insecure. Nursing education and service can combine forces to integrate their efforts as one means of enhancing the new graduates' transition from the student setting to the "real world" work situation.

Medical treatments, the coronary care unit, open heart surgery, cardiopulmonary resuscitation and even the complexities of today's intravenous solutions were unheard of 25 years ago. In the past several decades we have witnessed technological advances that have doubled, tripled and sometimes increased by exponential proportions the amount of knowledge that we expect our new nurse graduates to possess. At the same time, pressure from accrediting bodies, budgetary restrictions, lack of sufficient clinical facilities and the demands made by students themselves have forced educational agencies to reexamine their programs and selectively limit the amount of time spent in both didactic instruction and the actual practice of perfecting clinical skills. And as if this challenge were not of sufficient concern in terms of delineating nursing content, we are now faced with the added dimension of emerging roles for nurses—those roles which focus on the maintenance of health and prevention of illness.

In this era of "too much to learn and not enough time to learn it," it becomes apparent that educational programs cannot expect to prepare their graduates for all the contingencies of clinical practice. With this assumption, it becomes imperative that nursing educators and service administrators collectively examine and delineate the nature of learning experiences—(1) those that rightfully belong in educational programs and (2) those that would most logically become the responsibility of the service agencies. The need for a system which coordinates the efforts of these two groups would probably not have arisen during that period in nursing history when the hat of the nursing service director and the director of nursing education was donned by the same individual. Hence, in a way, such an effort would mean moving backward in history to reinstitute a theoretical model which again utilizes the input and services of both groups.

Preparing the Student for Graduation

The joint efforts of education and service are needed so that the transition from student to graduate is not an abrupt occurrence. In preparing for this transition, educators need to plan and provide experiences that introduce students to the realities of practice long before the day of graduation, and the employing service agencies in the community, in turn, must become familiar with and capitalize on these experiences as they assist the new graduate in adjusting to the work environment.

In an effort to prepare students for the realities of practice, the curricula in schools of nursing need to include learning experiences which are designed to provide for a maximum of self-direction and self-awareness. Such experiences will enable students to think and react appropriately in the type of problem situations that they are likely to encounter later in their experiences as graduate practitioners. Nursing instructors also need to focus on the realities of practice when planning clinical assignments. The "one nurse, one patient" concept is hardly a reality in the real world of nursing. The realities of practice also require that students become involved in day-to-day activities of the unit—assisting with passing trays when staffing on the unit is short—or being assigned to assist staff nurses who are clinically proficient.

Kramer has attributed the new graduates' lack of self-confidence to a "lack of 'interpersonal competency' which comes through to others and self as a lack of confidence."[1] Kramer goes on to explain that the lack of "interpersonal competency" arises when two sets of values are operative—those that the new graduate gained from the educational system and those that exist in the new work situation.[2] In

In an effort to prepare students for the realities of practice, the curricula in schools of nursing need to include learning experiences which are designed to provide for a maximum of self-direction and self-awareness.

such a setting, new graduates are unable to predict with any degree of accuracy the impact that their behavior will have upon others, or that the behavior of others will have upon them.

The lack of "interpersonal competency" is undoubtedly augmented by a perceived lack of confidence in the areas of skills, routines and other types of job-specific behaviors. It is a paradox in which the new graduate expounds with idealism about the profession and its future, while expressing feelings of personal inadequacy. It is as if the real world does not measure up to graduates' ideals; and they in turn are not prepared to function in the real world. With this dichotomy of ideals, it seems imperative that we help the new graduates sort out what they do know, assist them to apply this knowledge and motivate them to build on what they already know. In actual practice, most of the problems encountered in the clinical setting really do not require an on-the-spot decision or action anyway. It is usually possible to recognize a problem, study it and then act.

Educators must also be prepared to accept the responsibility for instilling in students the need to become lifelong learners, eager to participate in orientation and continuing education programs, and to be individuals responsible for their own continued development as nurses. Service agencies must then learn to utilize the new graduates' perception of themselves as lifelong learners as one means of helping them to overcome their lack of confidence.

Not only must we prepare students to perceive themselves as lifelong learners; but we must also develop informational programs which focus on educating employers, physicians, other staff nurses and health care workers in terms of the types and levels of competencies that can rightfully be expected of the new graduate. After all, we would not expect a new medical school graduate to be an accomplished internist or surgeon. In fact, most of the other health care professions—medicine, pharmacy, medical technology, etc.—include as part of their educational process an internship program.

Selecting Student Learning Experiences

With each advance in medical science has come a growing appreciation for one of the more costly elements of education, namely, time to learn the new content. With time as the scarce commodity, it becomes necessary for educational programs to differentiate between what is "nice to know and what is really essential." In this respect educational programs will need to consider for inclusion in their program and course objectives those cognitive, affective and psychomotor behaviors that are common to many areas of specialty practice. This implies the teaching of basic principles and concepts, rather than the teaching of specific facts and procedures which are easily forgotten.

As an example, students who have mastered the anatomy and physiology of the genitourinary system along with the principles of asepsis are less likely to have problems in catheterizing a patient in a new situation than will nurses who have simply committed to rote memory the basic steps of a procedure used for catheterizing a patient. Furthermore, the knowledge of anatomy and physiology can be applied to other situations, as can the understanding of asepsis. (See Figure 2.)

In terms of the time required for learning, it is only logical that educational programs should consider for inclusion in their programs those types of competencies—judgment skills, for example—that take a long time to master, or that require a student to move through a series of sequential steps to perfect. Service agencies, on the other hand, would probably find it more efficient in terms of time and funding to conduct programs aimed at teaching those skills which take relatively little time to learn, or which differ from agency to agency.

FIGURE 2. DECISION-MAKING MODEL FOR SELECTION OF CURRICULUM CONTENT

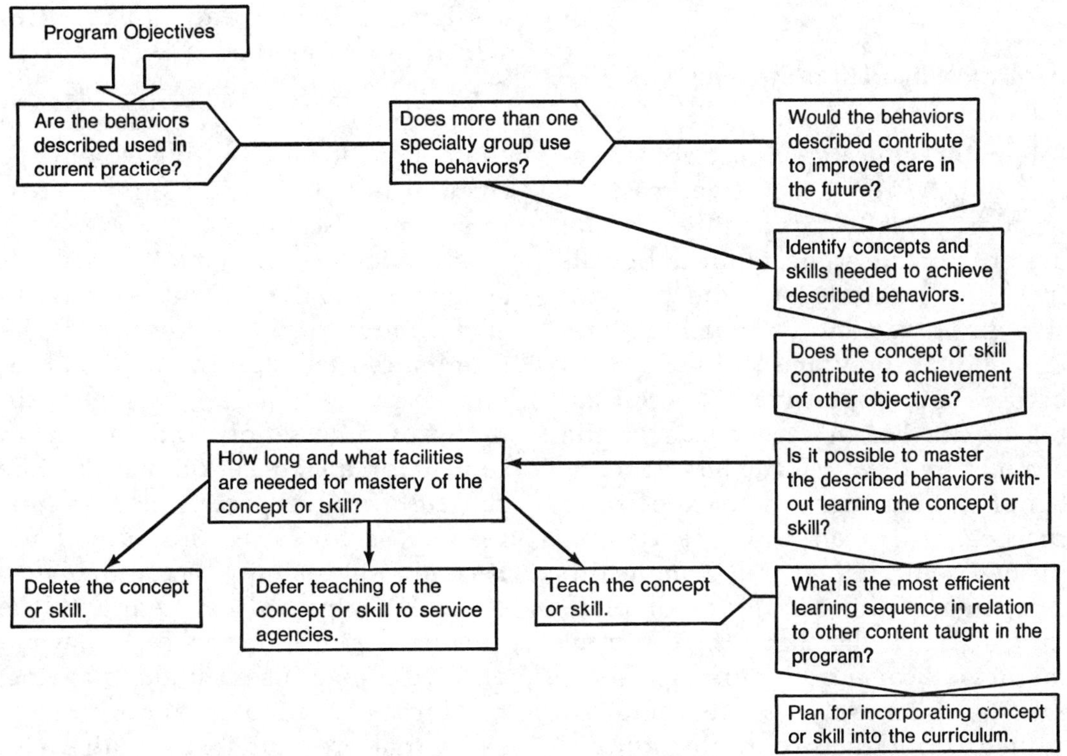

Specialization in the area of health care suggests a need to offer elective courses in the specialty areas of practice—geriatrics, coronary care and community health nursing, for example. These offerings would provide students with an opportunity to gain additional knowledge and experience in an area of practice which is particularly meaningful to them because it can be related to their specific career goals. Elective courses would also reduce the amount of inservice education that must be assumed by service agencies. It is even possible that the offering of elective courses will encourage students to begin identifying specific career goals at an earlier point in their educational program.

Accountability Both to Nursing and to Students

Nursing education must accept responsibility for keeping abreast of what is actually happening on the current nursing scene, while anticipating changes needed for the progressive improvement in nursing care. Educational programs will need to become both responsive and accountable to the health care needs of the community in which the largest number of its graduates can be expected to practice. This can only be accomplished by utilizing input from health care organizations in terms of planning for curricular changes. This input might well come from nursing leaders in the community, or it could be gained through survey techniques which serve to collect data from representative health care agencies in the community.

There are other means to insure that content taught in nursing programs is appropriate. Such means focus on the interaction between education and service personnel. In this respect, nursing educators might serve as employees and/or consultants for service agencies; while nursing service personnel could be given dual appointments where they have responsibility to the school of nursing for teaching students, and to the community agency for providing patient care. Small towns and rural areas might investigate bringing nurse educators into their communities during periods of time in which classes are not in session. Colleges and universities which supply graduates to these communities might even welcome the opportunity to bring students into these areas for an elective experience in rural nursing during spring recess or summer vacation.

Educational programs have a responsibility to the student as well as to the community. In terms of the economics of education, students today make a sizable investment in terms of time, effort and money in return for an education which they can rightfully expect to use. In this respect, schools of nursing must become increasingly accountable to students for providing them with the quality of education to which they are entitled. Programs must guard against producing graduates who possess skills that are outdated or otherwise unmarketable. As McMullen points out, "nursing education must see itself as not only accountable for providing students with the quality of education to which they are entitled, but also to the kind of education that will prepare them to meet people's health and nursing needs."[3]

In terms of time, educational programs will need to examine the flexibility that is afforded individual students as they progress through the program. For the most part, students come to the educational setting from a variety of backgrounds and with a variety of experiences. It seems foolhardy to require a student who has, for example, mastered the skills of bathing and bed making through prior experience as a nursing assistant to spend an equal amount of time, or even go through the same learning activities as the student who has not had the same experiences. There is a need to develop measurement tools which evaluate previous learning and which allow students to bypass learning activities that require merely an input of time,but that produce no new learning.

There is a need to develop measurement tools which evaluate previous learning and which allow students to bypass learning activities that require merely an input of time, but that produce no new learning.

The need to establish goals to which both nursing service and education can subscribe emphasizes the necessity for continued dialogue between the two groups. As nursing professionals concerned with the delivery of quality patient care, the two groups must come together to identify and describe common problems, to discuss the limitation imposed on each other, and come to some common understanding. In this respect, faculty from schools of nursing will need to do more than teach students; they will need to spend time in community health care facilities observing the use of and testing the knowledge that is presented in the classroom. After all, the clinical setting still remains the proving ground for the testing of nursing knowledge—or truth is what works.

REFERENCES

1. Kramer, M. *Reality Shock: Why Nurses Leave Nursing* (St. Louis: The C.V. Mosby Co. 1974) p. 29.
2. Ibid. p. 30–31.
3. McMullen, D. "Accountability and Nursing Education." *Nursing Outlook* 23:8 (1975) p. 502.

SUGGESTED READING

Vogelberger, M. "The Professional Adjustment and Growth of the New Graduate." *The Journal of Continuing Education* 2:5 (September-October 1971) p. 21–27.

Carol M. Porth, R.N., M.S.N., Ph.D.
Instructor
Education Department
Family Hospital
Associate Professor
School of Nursing
University of Wisconsin-Milwaukee
Milwaukee, Wisconsin

EASING THE TRANSITION FROM CLASSROOM INTO CLINICAL SETTING—IMPLICATIONS FOR SERVICE

Kramer documents the shock-like turmoil new graduates often encounter in the first year of employment.[1] Health care agencies have also felt the result of "reality shock" as turnover rates have increased and self-actualization through job satisfaction has diminished.

Administrators, realizing that the new graduate needs a period of adjustment following graduation, have supported programs that enable new graduates to make the transition from student to professional practitioner. At Family Hospital this need was recognized in early 1974. The Education Department was given the task of developing a program for new graduates that would enable them to make this transition through support and guidance.

Before establishing the Nurse Internship Program at Family, Nursing Service and the Education Department examined the curriculum of the associate degree, diploma and baccalaureate programs in the Milwaukee area. Although we have since employed a large number of graduates from programs outside the immediate area, initial recruitment efforts were directed toward schools in the immediate vicinity.

The adjustments new graduates make immediately after employment had been documented by Kramer and others. Literature showed that other acute care settings recognized the need to develop nurse internship programs. Discussions with new graduates presently in the setting helped to determine some adjustment factors they faced upon employment.

The first adjustment new graduates make is often to the acute care setting itself. Nursing, which has been the main focus in preparatory education, now becomes a part of the whole network of activity that is defined as the delivery of health care. This, coupled with the fact that new graduates usually have not established a level of expertise within their own discipline can make the initial adjustment difficult.

When graduates are adjusting to the acute care setting, the hospital often takes on the character of "the establishment." Graduate nurses often come from the free thinking, "ivory tower existence of academia" where they have not been held down by structured commitment. Working 40 hours a week, punching in and out and relying on someone else to determine time schedules can be a tremendous adjustment for the new nurse both physically and mentally.

Adjustment of new graduates to a professional role involves several factors. New graduates assume the same responsibility as an RN the day they begin employment. Throughout the education program, patient care is centered around one to two patients and seldom for an eight-hour period of time. Nursing instructors are visibly present, evaluating nursing care plans, explaining the relationship of physiology and disease process, and often accompanying students when they perform procedures. New graduates now face the prospect of taking care of larger numbers of patients, being responsible for activities such as change of shift report and telephone orders, making independent clinical judgments and being responsible not only for their own activities, but in many instances accountable for the level of care given by others.

This adjustment to the professional role is influenced by the relationship new graduates must develop with the other health care disciplines. This is especially true of their relationships with physicians. Seldom have new graduates in their student days perceived the subtleties of the "doctor-nurse game" they now must master to exist in a bureaucratic setting.

Another adjustment to consider is the relationship new graduates will have to develop with a different set of colleagues. In school, students have the luxury of often being at the same level of development as their peers. In a hospital setting, new graduates must establish a working relationship with other professional nurses who may differ in levels of experience and educational preparation. The beginning commonality is gone. Expectations the nursing staff may have of new graduates, coupled with the increased anxiety level of the new nurses, can polarize relationships from the very beginning.

Finally, the adjustment some new graduates have to make is with nursing itself. As one recent graduate stated, "I don't really know if I want to be a nurse." As uncomfortable as this may be to hear, for a small number of new graduates it is a factor that influences their adjustment to nursing practice.

Realizing the factors of adjustment that influence nurses as they enter the work environment, the Nurse Internship Program was developed. We have defined it as a three-month program that facilitates the integration of graduate nurses into the hospital setting through support, increased knowledge and opportunity to practice. The components of the Internship Program are identified as: (1) a well-defined *support system* to make the transition period easier, (2) relevant class discussions to build upon existing knowledge and increase awareness of capabilities and job function and (3) clinical experience to increase expertise of nursing practice.

The components of the Family Hospital Internship Program include relevant class discussions to build upon existing knowledge and increase awareness of capabilities and job function, and clinical experience to increase expertise of nursing practice.

The Support System

The support system of the Internship Program begins at the administrative level. The board of directors, hospital administrators, the director of nursing service and the hospital education department must share the belief that an internship program is necessary. They must also realize that the success of the internship is contingent upon the ability of each program to individualize itself to the needs of the institution and participating graduates.

The role of the internship coordinator is vital in developing and maintaining a support system for new graduates or "nurse interns" as we identify them at Family Hospital.

Support is initiated by having one person responsible for planning, evaluating and coordinating the three-month program. Since all disciplines and departments are involved with new employees, the goals and objectives of the internship must be shared by the coordinator. In order to elicit participation and support, a sound working relationship with hospital staff must be maintained.

The role of the coordinator is to facilitate, guide and provide resources to nurse interns. The coordinator must be clinically competent and available to new graduates throughout the program. It is important that the coordinator maintain the same schedule as the interns, including evening, night and weekend rotation.

The coordinator need not become a surrogate instructor. The interns must learn to identify their own learning needs while becoming autonomous practitioners. They must increase their skills for self-directed learning and develop an attitude for lifelong learning. However, it is the coordinator who reinforces these behaviors and guides new graduates through appropriate learning activities.

The coordinator should be cognizant of the adjustments new graduates must make with the initial employment and of the strengths they bring to the institution. It is also essential that the coordinator assess the positives and negatives that exist in the work setting and be able to deal with both sides in a realistic way.

The support system is further developed through participation of the staff on each unit. Unit staff function as clinical resources and behavior models. Staff with a good perception of what faces nurse interns when they begin employment are invaluable in helping new graduates in role identification and integration into the total work setting.

The interns themselves provide the final link in the support system. Weekly conferences are held, giving new graduates the opportunity to share feelings and experiences. Although the conferences are guided by the internship coordinator, discussion allows for peer identification of common role adjustments.

Class Discussion

Classes offered during the internship should build upon existing knowledge. Our experience has proven that it is best to offer classes concentrated into one full day or one half day each week. This allows interns to remain on the unit for a full shift.

Content for class presentation should reflect the learning needs of the interns. This will vary with the composition of the group and needs to be reevaluated throughout the program.

Skill and procedural classes have proven beneficial, since lack of nursing skills is a common problem experienced by nurse interns. Hospital policy can easily be incorporated into class content. Personnel from each department and discipline acquaint the interns with their activities. This allows each discipline to share its area of expertise and demonstrate to the interns the multidisciplinary approach necessary for patient care. Role playing, case studies and mock assignments are methods that have been used to teach patient care management, personal organization and priority-setting skills.

Clinical Experience

The main focus of the Internship Program is on clinical practice. The length of the program has proven adequate in increasing interns' clinical skills, adjusting to the work environment and developing confidence in practice and judgment.

Nurse interns are on the clinical unit for a full shift, four days per week. Because it is essential to provide a realistic experience, nurse interns are given the opportunity to work all three shifts and some weekends with the internship coordinator available.

The focus of the clinical experience is skill mastery, patient care management and clinical judgment making. Patient assignment reflects the learning needs of the nurse intern. The initial assignment may be two patients so that opportunity is given to practice skills in nursing procedures. As the intern gains experience, patient load is gradually increased so that the intern gains confidence in the organization skills necessary for delivery of care to larger groups of patients. By the final two weeks of the program, the nurse intern carries a full patient assignment.

Most clinical experience is gained on the unit where interns will be working after completion of the program. During the 12-week program, the interns are provided with the opportunity to rotate, for observational experience, to other areas of the hospital such as surgery, recovery room, outpatient and the intensive care unit.

During the last month of the internship, interns are placed on a "sister unit" for one week. For example, if an intern has been working on a medical floor, he or she will be assigned to a surgical floor. Through this experience interns can increase skill proficiency and broaden their understanding of the total delivery of health care.

Developing a transitional program for graduate nurses entering an acute care setting does not erase the chasm that presently exists between education and service. This dilemma needs to be seriously evaluated. Both sides must feel responsibility, not only for the educational preparation of beginning practitioners, but for the quality of patient care that is rendered in health care institutions.

Although a nurse internship program is not the total answer to this problem, such a transitional orientation program can provide realistic support of new graduates as they become integrated into the reality of the work setting.

REFERENCE

1. Kramer, M. *Reality Shock: Why Nurses Leave Nursing* (St. Louis: The C.V. Mosby Co. 1974).

SUGGESTED READINGS

Fleming, B., Woodstock, A. and Boyd, B. "A Nurse Internship Program." *American Journal of Nursing* 75:4 (April 1975) p. 595–599.

Martel, G. and Edmunds, M. "Nurse Internship Program in Chicago." *American Journal of Nursing* 72:5 (May 1972) p. 940–943.

McCloskey, J. "What Rewards Will Keep Nurses on the Job?" *American Journal of Nursing* 75:4 (April 1975) p. 600–602.

Schmalenberg, C. and Kramer, M. "Dreams and Reality: Where Do They Meet?" *The Journal of Nursing Administration* 6:6 (June 1976) p. 35–43.

Treece, E. *Internship in Nursing Education: Technoterm* (New York: Springer Publishing Co. 1974).

Mary E. Cramer, R.N., B.S.N.
Director of Staff Development
Ohio State University
Columbus, Ohio
Former Internship Coordinator
Family Hospital
Milwaukee, Wisconsin

CONTINUING EDUCATION

Evaluating Continuing Education: Quantification or Involvement?

Donald A. Bille, R.N., Ph.D.
Associate Professor
Department of Nursing
DePaul University
Chicago, Illinois
Former Assistant Professor
Nursing Service Administration
College of Nursing
University of Illinois at the Medical Center
Chicago, Illinois

Maureen Fitzgibbons, R.N., B.S.N.
Clinical Instructor
Department of Nursing Education and Research
Mercy Hospital and Medical Center
Chicago, Illinois

"Well, in our country," said Alice, still panting a little, "you'd generally get to somewhere else—if you ran very fast for a long time, as we've been doing."

"A slow sort of country!" said the Queen. "Now, here you see, it takes all the running you can do, to keep in the same place. If you want to get somewhere else, you must run at least twice as fast as that!"

Through the Looking-Glass
Lewis E. Carroll

PROFESSIONAL NURSES of the 70s are facing the same sort of dilemma that Alice faced. It takes all the running we can do to be nurses, but it takes even more running to keep up with today's ever-expanding knowledge and technology. Continuing Education (CE) plays an important role in the health care industry by helping nurses "run at least twice as fast" to improve their knowledge, understanding, skills, atti-

The authors wish to thank the staff nurses of Mercy Hospital and Medical Center, Chicago, Illinois, who participated on the patient teaching workshop committee.

tudes, values and interests; and by preparing nurses for an expanded role.[1]

The need for continuing education has been recognized since about the turn of the century. ". . . There must be provided means by which the women may keep in touch with new lines of research in medicine and methods in nursing."[2] In addition to this early recognition of the need for continuing nursing education, early adult educators recognized the fact that "if you bring nurses back for continuation training, you will have to accumulate something which it will be profitable for them to study when they arrive."[3]

Is CE profitable? Are continuing nursing education programs working? Many people are asking these questions and educators, in turn, are asking "How can I prove that CE has made a difference? How can I tell if it did what I wanted it to do?"

THE NEED FOR EVALUATING CE

A cursory perusal of CE literature over the past few years reveals repeated calls for a means to evaluate the outcome of CE. But to date, there is little help or direction available for evaluating CE. Educators are confused when they have to demonstrate what the outcome of their workshops are. It would be ideal if we could demonstrate with sound, hard data (which has statistical significance) that our programming has achieved changes in behavior. But this hard data may be hard to get.

Miller states that, at times, "finding ways of measuring progress demands more technical resources than we often have available."[4] Knowles lists four factors which limit the ability to properly evaluate learning outcomes:

- Human behavior is too complex to prove what changed it.
- Changes that occur after a workshop are not always measurable (with current instruments).
- Evaluation can be very expensive, especially in time investments.
- Participation is still primarily voluntary (so program worth can be tested by participant satisfaction).[5]

How, then, do we measure progress? There are two approaches to education which must be considered in order to evaluate its effectiveness—the content oriented approach and the involvement approach.

The Content Oriented Approach

Content oriented education gives primary importance to content dissemination, where the teacher imparts facts and information to the students. In a purely content oriented approach to education, the learner's head is perceived as having a hole in it, into which the teacher pours facts. Postman and Weingartner describe the teacher as a lamplighter who penetrates the darkness and illuminates the learner's mind, or the gardener who cultivates the mind, providing fertilizer so that seeds of knowledge will grow. Then there is the personnel manager who keeps the students' minds busy, making them efficient and industrious; the muscle builder who strengthens flabby minds; the bucket filler who fills them up;[6] and the banker who deposits knowledge in the minds of the students.[7]

According to the content approach, the teacher's role is to cram into the student as many facts as possible in the time allotted, giving students a strange resemblance to "Belgian geese being fattened for pate de foie gras."[8]

Progress in content oriented education can be determined by measuring the amount of information transmitted from teacher to student. Evaluation of this approach would be greatly concerned with efficiency—with getting data which determines whether or not the teacher is producing maximum change in the shortest possible time at the least cost—that is, quantification.[9]

The Involvement Approach

The involvement approach to education regards teachers as the **facilitators** of learning, since they facilitate self-development and provide resources for the students' self-directed inquiry. Under this approach, the teachers (facilitators) are more concerned with the relationship between themselves and the learners,[10] and the learning process is more important than the amount of information transmitted.

Knowles said, the teacher "incurs an obligation to involve the participants in collecting data that will enable them to assess the effectiveness of the program in helping them accomplish their objectives. His dominant theme will be involvement."[11]

QUANTIFICATION OR INVOLVEMENT?

Is the process of continuing nursing education one which can be **quantified,** or should its merits be determined on the basis of **involvement?**

The Department of Nursing Education and Research, which evaluated a continuing nursing education workshop titled "Patient Teaching: a Multidisciplinary Approach," believed that by involving the participants in their own evaluation, they could learn to get evidence for themselves about the progress they were making toward their own goals. Their decision to use the involvement approach was based on the proposition that there is a unique technology of adult education (Andragogy) which makes certain assumptions about the unique characteristics of adults as learners.

During the evaluation, a representative group of staff nurses assisted in a problem census concerning patient teaching activities. Two productive meetings were held which identified the following objectives:

1. At the end of the workshop, the participant would be able to recognize that patient education is an essential component of comprehensive patient care; to delineate factors which influence patient education; to outline principles of adult education as related to patient education; to discuss the medical-legal aspects

of patient education; and to demonstrate a means of documentation of patient education.

2. In a guided work session, the participant will be able to formulate a patient teaching plan.

The objectives would be accomplished in an all day workshop, divided into nine different parts (see Appendix A), the last of which was a guided self-evaluation (see Appendices B and C).

Self-Evaluation

The guided self-evaluation was to be accomplished approximately one month after attending the patient teaching workshop. The self-evaluation requests the participants to think back to the workshop (which encourages retention of the learned material) and state something about what (how much) was learned. It also asks participants to describe how their practice had changed, as well as what concepts they intended to utilize but had not yet done so (which stimulates self-motivation for trying out the new concepts). Finally, the self-evaluation guide asked participants to identify further needs for CE in the area of patient teaching (as a means of future program planning). (See Appendix A). To ensure full participation, participants were required to submit their completed self-evaluations before receiving a certificate of attendance from the workshop. (Participants were granted one contact hour for this self-evaluation.)

The results of the self-evaluations gave the workshop leaders an idea of how well the program's objectives were met (how much was learned), and to what extent. The results also indicated that professional nurses, given guidance through CE, can take responsibility not only for deciding what patient care values they have, what their goals are and the extent to which they have achieved their goals, but also they will have learned to take responsibility for their own learning and the direction their patient care will take.

Developing an Internal Sense through Involvement

Through involvement in the continuing nursing education process, learners do not need external evaluation, or quantification; they develop an **internal sense** of how they compare to how they would like to be. This same internal sense becomes a motivational drive towards closing the gap between what is and what should be. It may help nurses "run at least twice as fast" in order to "get somewhere else!"

Through involvement in the continuing nursing education process, learners . . . develop an* internal sense *of how they compare to how they would like to be. This same internal sense becomes a motivational drive towards closing the gap between what is and what should be.

REFERENCES

1. Spector, A. "The ANA and Continuing Education." *Journal of Continuing Education in Nursing* 2 (March–April 1971) p. 45.
2. Editorial. *The American Journal of Nursing* 3 (May 1903) p. 668.
3. Judd, C. H. "Adult Education." *The American Journal of Nursing* 28 (July 1928) p. 654–655.
4. Miller, H. L. *Teaching and Learning in Adult Education* (New York: MacMillan Co. 1964) p. 294.
5. Knowles, M. S. *The Modern Practice of Adult Education: Andragogy versus Pedagogy* (New York: Association Press 1970) p. 220.
6. Postman, N. and Weingartner, C. *Teaching as a Subversive Activity* (New York: Delacourt Press 1969) p. 82.
7. Freire, P. *Pedagogy of the Oppressed* (New York: Herder and Herder 1972) p. 58.
8. Miller, G. E. "Adventure in Pedagogy." *Journal of the American Medical Association* 162 (December 15, 1956) p. 1448.
9. Knowles. *Modern Practice.* p 222.
10. Rogers, C. *Freedom to Learn* (Columbus, Ohio: Charles E. Merrill Co. 1969) p. 106.
11. Knowles. *Modern Practice.* p. 222.

Appendix A
Patient Teaching Workshop

I. INTRODUCTION (15 Minutes)

This short session will set the stage for the conference. Through use of a slide-sound presentation, the participant will experience the emotions of a patient who is admitted to the hospital and not given the appropriate orientation to his surroundings. The objectives of the workshop will then be presented to the group.

II. NEED FOR PATIENT EDUCATION (30 Minutes)

Using an historical survey of literature, the concept of patient teaching will be developed as an integral part of comprehensive nursing care. Participants will be brought up to date on standards and guidelines for patient teaching set forth by ANA, JCAH, and other organizations such as the American Hospital Association (AHA). One sample of philosophy of patient teaching will be developed during this hour.

III. PRINCIPLES OF ADULT EDUCATION RELATED TO PATIENT TEACHING (3 Hours)

The theory of "Andragogy" will be presented and related to the process of teaching the hospitalized adult. Through lecture, discussion, and a question-and-answer session, participants will be exposed to teaching-learning theory, requirements which must be present in order to learn, the nursing process as one means of planning an educational experience, and methods of evaluation of patient teaching-learning.

IV. MEDICAL-LEGAL ASPECTS OF PATIENT EDUCATION (30 Minutes)

A lecture and question-and-answer period will deal with an interpretation of the new Illinois Nurse Practice Act, and within this parameter the possible pitfalls and potentials for malpractice in patient teaching will be developed.

V. DOCUMENTATION (1 Hour)

Through lecture, demonstration, and case study, the documentation of patient learning will be presented and practiced. Assessment of patient's knowledge, teaching efforts, and evidence of learning will be dealt with.

VI. WORK SESSION (1 Hour)

The participants will be arranged in small groups and guided through an experience in which they will plan a teaching program for a given disease or condition. Resource material will be provided in the classroom as a means of establishing and validating the material to be given to the patients. Evaluation of participants' learning will be judged by their ability to write objectives, arrive at a means of assessing prior knowledge, plan teaching methodology, and plan several evaluation questions.

VII. QUESTION AND ANSWER PERIOD (30 Minutes)

VIII. EVALUATION OF WORKSHOP (15 Minutes)

IX. EVALUATION OF PERFORMANCE

One month after the workshop, the participants will be asked to complete a second evaluation, in which they evaluate their own performance as a result of attendance at the workshop.

Appendix B
Post-Workshop Self-Evaluation

About one month ago, you attended a workshop on Principles of Patient Teaching. Please answer the following questions as honestly as you can, then evaluate your own practice and decide where change is needed.

1. What concepts do you remember learning about patient teaching as the result of this workshop.

____

____

____

2. Which concepts, presented at the workshop, have you already put to use in your own care.

____

____

____

3. Which concepts, presented at the workshop, have you *not* been able to implement? (Please site example and possible reason why.)

____

____

____

4. Which concepts do you still intend to try to implement in providing care.

____

____

____

5. Do you have a need for more continuing education in the area of patient teaching? If yes, what do you need? (Communicate these needs to your Inservice Department).

____

____

____

____

Appendix C
Self-Evaluation Checklist

1. Indicate how much you feel you learned:
   —Importance of documentation.
   —Medical-legal aspects.
   —Importance of patient teaching.
   —Five basic steps in teaching-learning process.
   —Right to informed consent.
   —Use of behavioral objectives.
   —How to recognize teachable moment.
   —Importance of assessment.
   —Importance of organized teaching plan.
   —Evaluation of patient's learning.
   —Teaching can be both formal and informal.
   —Importance of individual approach to each patient.
   —Realizing our responsibility was so great.
   —Importance of realistic objectives.
   —Should be geared to individual needs and abilities.
   —Keep language as simple as possible.
   —Dealing with denial.
   —Ideas for approaching patients.
   —New concepts for implementation of teaching.
   —Brought many concepts together.
   —Teaching as a means of encouraging better self-care.
   —Patient's participation aids in decreasing anxiety.

2. Which concepts have you put to use in your nursing care:
   —Documentation of teaching.
   —Assessment of learning needs.
   —Identifying needs, forming objectives, methods to achieve objectives.
   —More specific, measurable, realistic teaching plans.
   —Discharge needs.
   —Evaluation tools.
   —Five basic steps of teaching-learning process.
   —Reinforcement of learning.
   —Awareness of teaching opportunities.
   —Need for compliance.
   —Return demonstration of skills.
   —Make teaching a part of every day nursing care.
   —Repetition increases retention of learnings.
   —Implementation of teaching objectives.
   —Preventative teaching.
   —Communication techniques—create climate of trust.
   —Group teaching techniques.

3. Which concepts have you *not* been able to implement:
   —Evaluation of learning.
   —Need for documentation of teaching.
   —Discharge teaching.
   —Family involvement.
   —Concise charting.
   —Concise teaching plan.
   —Better nurse-physician communication.
   —More continuity of care.
   —Reinforcement.
   —Discharge planning.
   —Admission assessment.
   —Formal classes for similar patients' diagnoses.
   —Assessment of readiness to learn.

—Better care plans.
—Treat each patient individually.
—File of teaching cards for common, easy to understand procedures.
—Importance of compliance to avoid rehospitalization.
—Utilization of every nursing task as teachable moment.
—Involvement of other health care team members.

4. Which concepts do you still intend to try to implement:
—Better documentation.
—Family involvement.
—Assessment of patients' readiness to learn.
—Evaluation of learning.
—Patients' right to information.
—Discharge planning.
—Teaching on a daily basis.
—Reinforcement of learning.
—Teaching formula or method.
—Continuity in teaching.
—New teaching techniques.
—Assessment of existing knowledge.
—More realistic objectives.
—Writing goals for patient teaching.
—Post-hospitalization self-care.
—Improvement of nursing care plans.
—Interdepartmental communication.
—Post-hospitalization follow-up.
—Use daily routines as teaching moment.
—Teaching in understandable terms.
—More disease oriented programs like "Diabetes Teaching Program".
—Keep patient informed about procedures, tests and daily care routines.
—Health maintenance teaching.
—More regard for socioeconomic values.
—Improved interaction.

5. Need for more continuing education:
—Patient teaching regarding specific disease entities.
—Medical-legal aspects.
—Discharge planning.
—Audio-visual aids in patient teaching.
—Teaching methods.
—Documentation.
—Formulating objectives.
—Educational materials available for patient teaching.
—Outside resources.
—Family involvement.
—Motivation.
—Follow-up care.
—How to deal with the patient who refuses to learn.
—Assisting patient to deal with imposed changes in lifestyle.
—Pharmacology.
—Outpatient teaching.
—SOAP charting.
—Health maintenance.

Staff Development at University Hospital, University of Washington

THE DEPARTMENT OF NURSING SERVICES AND STAFF DEVELOPMENT: AN OVERVIEW

THE STAFF DEVELOPMENT program at University Hospital, University of Washington, Seattle, is inseparable from other parts of the Department of Nursing Services. It reflects and supports the department's overall philosophy, goals and activities.

In 1973, the nursing organization, under the progressive leadership of Ruth B. Fine, was given the opportunity to create the "ideal" nursing department. Members of the Executive Council had already determined that the traditional hierarchical organization was outdated. Furthermore, it was inconsistent with the high degree of professionalism, the highly complex role of the nursing staff and the flexibility demanded of a dynamic organization able to respond to the changing needs of the patient and society. Already the nursing department was highly participative, and new programs such as primary nursing were being initiated at the "grassroots" level. It seemed an ideal time for organizational change. We felt there might be a better way to structure the organization to support the staff nurse in providing quality patient care.

The Management Council, consisting of nurse coordinators (NCs), nursing administrative supervisors, clinical nurse specialists, assistant and associate directors of nursing, and the director of nursing, met for a day-long retreat with the overall objective of discussing creative plans which would support the nurse in providing quality patient care. The underlying concepts formed at this retreat remain the basis for the structure, planning and ongoing change occurring at University Hospital today. These concepts represent the philosophical and organizational basis for the direction of our educational programs.

Designing the Ideal Nursing Department

We determined to keep one organizing concept central to our discussions: the needs of the patient and the nurse caring for the patient would be the center of all reorganization planning. We began by looking at the needs of the patient, then at the needs of the nurse providing care to the patient, then at the nursing care delivery system that would best meet those needs. Only then did we begin to look at the unit structure and the total organizational structure. We wanted an organizational structure that centered around the needs of the patient and around the support systems needed for the nurse in providing care to the patient.

A second organizing concept was "accountability at all levels" of the organization. Such a concept is not new to nursing professionals, but we felt it a major component of the autonomy, expanded role and critical judgments we were expecting of the nursing staff. With the high degree of complexity of the organization and the high level of professional preparation among the nursing staff, we sought to structure the organization so that decision making would take place at the level closest to that of implementation. This would mean a high degree of autonomy for individuals making decisions for the patient, a high level of responsibility by each individual unit for their organizational milieu and patient care, and would require sophisticated skills in decision making, communication and group process. We felt, too, that those of us at the executive council level needed to demonstrate an accountability to the nursing units, to each other and to the organization that would be visible and measurable.

We wanted an organization that would provide optimal use of the education and expertise of all staff at all levels. We had then, and continue to have, only RNs (89 percent) and LPNs (11 percent) providing direct care to patients. We believed that support of the nurses in developing an autonomous, assertive and professional role would be basic to the full use of their education and skills, and could only result in positive outcomes for the patients. We saw primary nursing as one possible approach to meeting this goal, and determined to study it fully for possible wider implementation.

Similarly, we felt that each nursing unit would benefit from an organization in which members of the executive council were able to develop and utilize their special area of expertise, based on organizational need. Each individual staff nurse, and each unit should have access to any resource, depending on their need. By broad and flexible role definitions as opposed to narrow and restrictive role definitions, we could best support staff nurses in their expanding roles, and could best utilize each executive council member's skills and expertise to the fullest.

Building an organizational system around the needs of the nurse providing care to the patient, promoting accountability at all levels of the organization, decision making at the level closest to that of implementation, and maximum utilization of education and expertise of all staff at all levels were inconsistent with the role of the traditional supervisor. We decided to work toward elimination of the "supervisor" role, and instead build a group of "resource persons" who were highly skilled in areas representing the support needs of nursing staff and who could collectively provide support and guidance to the nursing units. This group of resources, representing expertise in patient care, staff development and management, would function on a matrix model, thereby meeting the need for flexibility in a complex and rapidly changing organization.

In order to match resources with needs, to make visible each person's role and area of accountability, and to provide a basis for evaluation, all members of the organization would enter into a contract with the organization, based on the organization's needs and on their individual areas of expertise, to be renegotiated yearly and as the needs of the organization changed. Contracts became another organizing concept.

In looking at the support needed by the nurse in providing care to the patient, a strongly identified need was the separation of direct from indirect patient care activities, and the relief of the nurse of as many of the indirect tasks as possible. The reorganization planning group was most interested in looking at the unit management concept as a possible approach.

Finally, the group identified education as a strong and essential element of such an "ideal" organization. They felt that educational support was essential to a dynamic, changing and flexible organization, and to the highly skilled professional nurse de-

---

Education is a strong and essential element of an "ideal" nursing department. . . . educational support is essential to a dynamic, changing and flexible organization, and to the highly skilled professional nurse demanded by the changed structure.

---

manded by the changed structure. As a first step, we felt a need to bring new staff to a high level of skill more quickly than we had in the past. To do this, it was imagined that we could capitalize on the experiences available in the entire organization rather than on one particular unit, and therefore could build breadth and depth of competence more quickly. The total hospital then was termed the "phantom unit" and the concept of a rapid, intense and highly mobile orientation utilizing experiences from multiple units was termed "phantom orientation." Staff in the unit have become known as "phantoms" much to their dismay or enjoyment, depending on their frame of reference. Indeed, we now have "phantom objectives," "phantom clinical supervision," "phantom hiring," etc. Nevertheless, the concept has turned out to be less "ghostlike" than the term.

Reorganization of the Nursing Department

How, then, did the original group see the organization structured? A model was developed showing two interlocking circles representing the nursing organization. (See Figure 1.) One circle represented the nursing unit and the other the "resource center." The resource center was to include people with skills in patient care, education and staff development, and management. It would also include audio-visual equipment, learning resources, patient education resources, a library and secretarial support. The NC would report directly to the director of nursing, as would members of the resource center. Those of us in the resource center would maintain a collaborative, supportive or consultant role with the units, depending on their need. Our model showed quality assurance as an overlapping responsibility between the nursing units and the resource center. Nursing audit and management audit would serve, through a "quality assurance board" to match resources with needs, the agreement to be consummated through the "contract."

The management council then wrote a charge to a reorganization steering committee:

- Establish priorities with timetables for the total plan (as presently conceived).
- Establish appropriate task forces to develop components of plans and timetables.
- Coordinate and supervise task forces.
- Receive and review materials of task forces.
- Communicate reports of task forces to appropriate other forces and concerned groups.
- Incorporate approved work of task forces into proposed plan.
- Recommend implementation of approved plans for trial and evaluation.
- Keep all members of the nursing department aware of all phases and activities of reorganization.

It then set criteria and qualifications for members of the reorganization steering committee and conducted an election for steering committee membership. Since the beginning of

FIGURE 1. CONCEPTUAL MODEL: REORGANIZATION OF THE DEPARTMENT OF NURSING

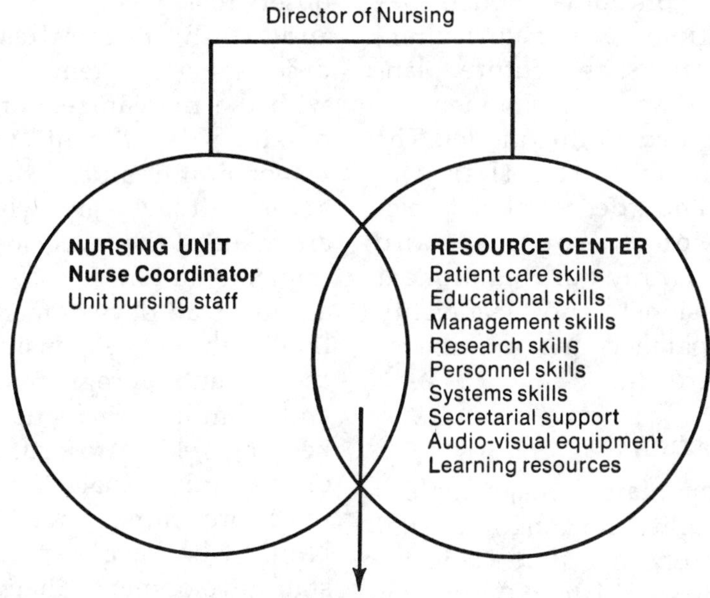

Overlapping Responsibilities

Quality assurance board
(matches resources with needs)
Contracts
Phantom unit (orientation)

Major Concepts

1. An organizational structure that best supports the nurse practitioner in providing optimal care to the patient.
2. Optimal use of education and expertise of all staff at all levels.
3. Focusing of expertise to the patient.
4. Implementation of primary nursing.
5. Decision making at the level closest to that of implementation of the decision.
6. Strong educational support for new and experienced staff.
7. Separation of nursing from nonnursing tasks.
8. Accountability of all nurses at all levels.
9. Contracts to be formally negotiated at all levels.

our reorganization program, the steering committee has developed charges to multiple task forces, and the job is not yet complete. Concepts such as primary nursing, contractual agreements, peer review, contractual staffing, systems, negotiated work load and resource center have become important parts of the overall reorganization process.

The Division of Staff Development utilizes a coordinated system of centralized and decentralized approaches to the staff development process. The overall program of the staff development division is tied together by a conceptual model. (See Figure 1.) Various parts of curriculum, ongoing programs and future planning for use and development of resources are tied to this model. The model also ties together the centralized and decentralized elements of our program, and demonstrates clearly our commitment to a professional and leadership growth that parallels and interrelates with clinical growth.

DECENTRALIZATION

Each unit maintains a major share of the responsibility for ongoing staff development on that unit. This arrangement is consistent with our philosophy of staff development, which states in part:

> We believe that recognition and utilization of individual potential occurs when staff members are involved in identifying their own learning needs and participate in planning ways of meeting these needs. Effective continuing education which results in visible improvement in patient care is dependent upon active participation of the staff.
>
> We believe that learning has taken place when a behavior change is evident in the learner. The value of that learning can be measured through observable changes in the patients and/or their families.

We feel our emphasis on decentralization is consistent with adult principles of learning, and that the opportunity to apply new learning based on a felt need, and to receive the immediate feedback available at the unit level is a system of organization that will most likely result in "an observable change in the patients and/or their families." Such a decentralized system is also consistent with the reorganized structure of the nursing department where strong responsibility and accountability rest at the unit level, and where decisions are made at the level closest to that of implementation. Each unit designates a "unit staff development representative" who is responsible for needs assessment, program development and planning, evaluation and record-keeping related to staff development on that unit. Usually these representatives are nurse practitioner IIs or NPIIIs who have a special interest in staff development. They combine this responsibility with their other patient care and leadership functions.

How then does the staff development division relate to the nursing unit? As a part of the resource center, members of the staff development division act as educational resources to the units in their development of educational programs. Our overall aim as a resource is to provide the educational expertise to enable each unit to develop an educationally effective staff development program, one with measurable objectives and outcomes that will mean a difference in patient care. As educational consultants, we facilitate, promote, participate in, advise or provide resources, depending on the unit need or readiness. Each unit, then, has one person from the staff development division who is their "staff development resource person."

CE REVAMPED

The educational programs at University Hospital developed centrally are those that are of a more universal need, and are designed to be ongoing and repetitive. They are approved for CE recognition points (CERPs) in the state of Washington. The leadership and management courses are an example of this aspect of our educational model. (See Figure 2.)

One way in which we combine and coordinate unit and central educational programs and in which we incorporate a **participative approach** to staff development with experiential learning for unit CE representatives is to develop a central educational offering planned by unit representatives with members of the staff development division acting as resources.

The staff development resource persons relate to the various members of the resource center in a collaborative and consultant role. For example, a major portion of the role of the clinical nurse specialist is in education. At times, resources from the staff development division may collaborate in the development of a particular program. At other times, we may be in a consultant role, and the clinical nurse specialists engage in multiple educational activities in which we play no active part. Our relationship depends on the need and objective of the particular program.

A similar flexible relationship exists between staff development resource persons and the various departmental committees and task forces. A member of the staff development division participates in each committee and task force. Though the entire committee remains responsible for the education related to its activities, the staff development resource persons may act as educational consultants. Likewise, they gain information about changes and planning that will influence the educational planning for the department. An important example of such involvement is with the nursing audit committee. Here, as in other committees, what is happening in the committee may influence the specific content of an orientation class, the currency and relatedness of the leadership program, or the need for educational planning. Such involvement assures programming, as well, that is consistent with the expected standards of clinical performance, that meets a genuine need, and supports the overall philosophy and direction of the nursing department.

The concepts basic to departmental reorganization are central to the educational program and planning, and are consistent with basic concepts of adult education. **Accountability** is a theme that influences our educational program at every level. It begins when the new orientee is asked to complete the nursing skills development worksheet. This tool is designed so that new staff persons determine their own learning needs, identify priorities, decide which learning resource will best meet their needs, and set a target date for completion. With assistance from an educational resource person, new staff members can develop individually planned

FIGURE 2. MODEL FOR STAFF DEVELOPMENT

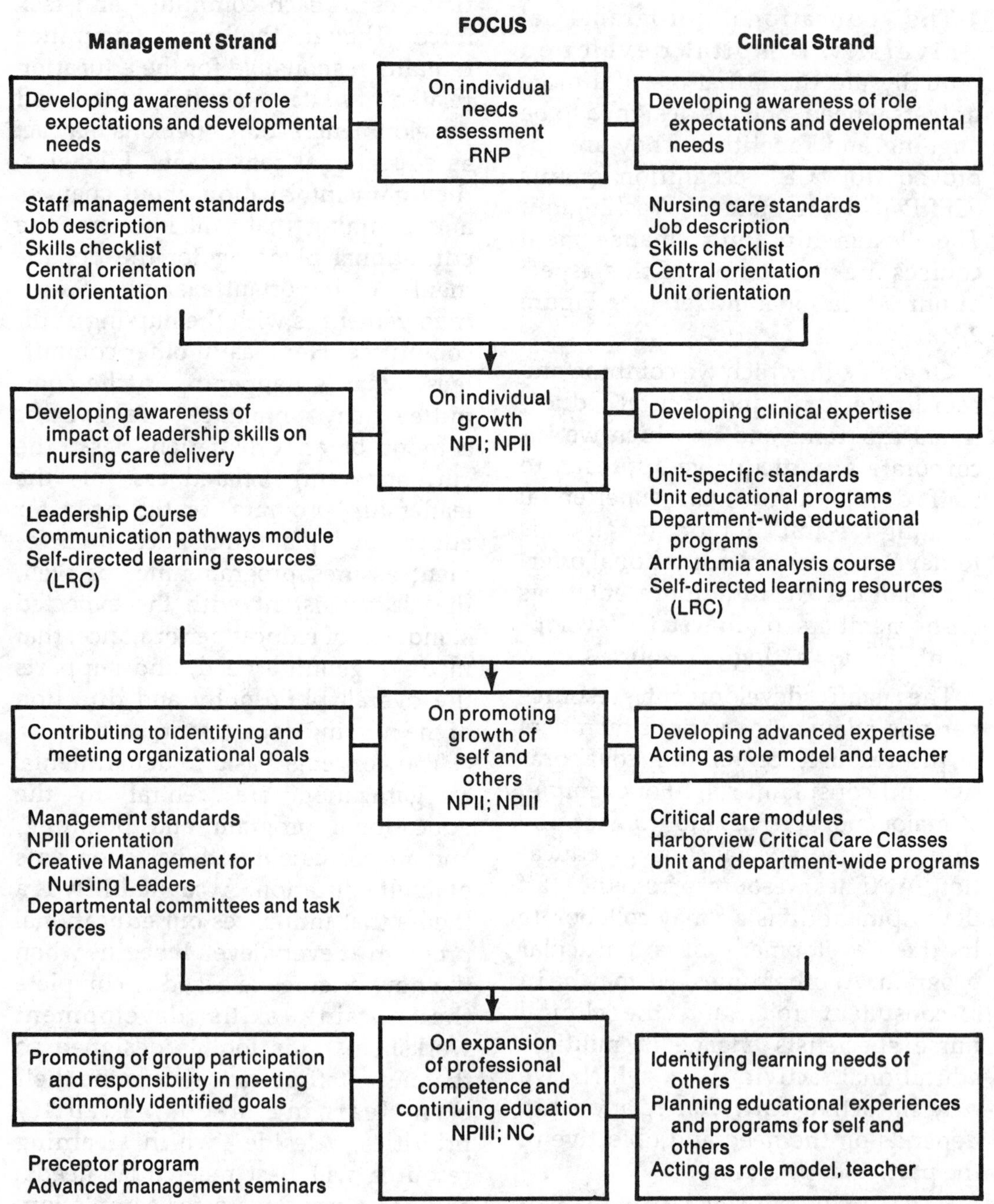

New staff nurses at University Hospital are accountable for their own continuing development, and this begins with their own individual identification of learning needs and planning.

learning pathways that will be consistent with their needs and the needs of the unit to which they will be assigned. New staff nurses, then, are accountable for their own continuing development, and this begins with their own individual identification of learning needs and planning.

The staff development division is in the process of building a learning resource center (LRC) designed to be consistent with the concept of accountability. It is planned to enable staff to be self-directed in finding and utilizing resources and learning experiences. Recognizing that staff come to the organization with differing knowledge, skill levels and learning needs, and that staff learn in a variety of different ways, we hope the center will provide the flexibility to learn in the way that best fits each staff member's learning style and needs.

Our emphasis on development and utilization of **self-directed learning** modules is consistent with self-directed and individualized learning. One of the first steps for our division was to develop standards, guidelines and resources for the development of learning modules. Once this was completed, we went about setting priorities for the development of modules for the areas of central orientation most conducive to self-directed learning. These areas were chosen from the nursing skills worksheet. These modules provide a means for pretesting knowledge and skill so learners can determine which objective they already meet, and can select a "learning tract," or the experience and resources, that will best meet their needs.

Many units, with the help of their staff development resource persons, are also developing learning modules that will be used in their orientation programs. These learning modules will enable new orientees to be self-directed and less dependent on an experienced staff member for their orientation. They will provide consistent information, with measurable outcomes, and will consume less time of unit nursing staff. One unit's hemovac learning module is one example. The critical care orientation program is also an example, representing multiple and reinforcing approaches to learning, enabling orientees to select their own pathways. Through a cooperative agreement with our sister university-managed hospital, Harborview Hospital, staff may attend critical care classes in their institution as one pathway in the module. Learning modules, then, provide another component of our education program that recognizes individuality and enhances accountability.

ACCOUNTABILITY AND EVALUATION

The staff development division is also trying to ensure its own accountability in a variety of ways. Overall, we feel an accountability to the consumer, so our programs are geared toward building an educational program that is measurable and positively affects the care the consumer receives, and that is cost-effective in terms of budget and in terms of the time staff spend away from direct patient care. So, we structured our central offerings so that behavioral change is measured. The staff development division, in an attempt to be accountable to the learner as well as to the patient, provides opportunities to evaluate the instructor for each centrally-prepared offering. Staff development resource persons are also attempting to assist unit CE representatives in building objectives and measurability into unit orientation and educational programs.

A sister tool to the nursing skills development worksheet is the yet-to-be developed "learning resource locator." The objective here, as with the skills development worksheet, is to provide a tool that will promote and enable individual staff accountability for their own development. The tool will also meet the need for visibility and accessibility of resources necessitated by the flattened organizational structure of reorganization. As the skills development worksheet is finalized, and as the system for cataloging and managing all available learning resources is completed, the learning resource locator will be developed. Staff members will be able to refer to the learning resource locator to determine: what resources are available related to a particular learning need; what type of resource it is, i.e., learning module, book or article, film, slide-tape presentation, videotape, regularly-offered class, etc.; and where the resource is located. The topics included will be consistent with the skills development worksheet. This tool, too, then is designed to enable the staff nurses to be accountable for their own learning.

IMPLEMENTATION OF PRIMARY NURSING

A major influence of reorganization on the staff development division's program has been the implementation of primary nursing. The leadership course was a direct result of the need to support professional nurses in their expanded role. Concepts that are key to primary nursing, such as *visible* accountability, defensible decision making, interpersonal effectiveness, assertiveness and intraprofessional respect and support, comprise the program core. This program had been particularly effective and well-received by the nursing staff.

CONTRACTING—A KEY CONCEPT OF REORGANIZATION

Contracting, another key concept of reorganization, is also a coordinating theme of the staff development division. It is, perhaps, demonstrated most graphically in the skills development worksheet. This is the new orientees' learning contract. It will identify to the orientee which parts of orientation are obligatory and which are self-directed. With their orientation instructor, orientees will determine which parts of the contract have priority, and will contract for study time, resource persons or experiences that will promote their learning program. Another example of a contract is the learning contract that participants in the leadership course sign. Such a contract emphasizes all participants' responsibility for their own learning, the necessity of their active participation in contributing to the group, and their responsibility for applying the concepts learned to their activity on the nursing unit.

Linda A. Kent, R.N., M.N.
Director, Nursing Staff Development
University Hospital

THE ROLE OF THE EDUCATIONAL CONSULTANT

The nursing services department is a decentralized organization designed to increase the quality of nursing care by establishing responsibility and accountability at every level. The problem-solving process in areas of management, patient care and staff development begins at the unit level, but involves other resource persons according to responsibility, involvement and expertise.

The staff development division places a major emphasis on staff development programs which assist nurses in recognizing and utilizing their individual potential. Every nurse is encouraged to actively participate in the learning process, however, each unit selects a staff development representative to coordinate unit staff development programs. Our division recognizes the need to assist these representatives, other nursing staff and NCS in developing quality programs which will result in visible improvement in patient care. Accordingly, each nursing unit is assigned an educational consultant from the staff development division. Consultants' degree of involvement with a unit will depend on the unit's readiness, the staff's perception of need, the educational consultants' overall time commitment, and their ability to make their expertise and the benefits of a well-planned educational offering visible to unit nursing staff.

The staff development division at University Hospital places a major emphasis on staff development programs which assist nurses in recognizing and utilizing their individual potential.

Planning

In the initial stages of planning, educational consultants may be asked to help identify learning needs of nursing staff. They may assist unit staff in conducting needs assessment or in performing task, performance or critical incident analysis. They may also encourage the use of other management level individuals or staff meetings in identifying learning needs.

Once learning needs are identified, consultants are in the position of helping staff to define sound learning objectives which will clearly describe desired behavioral outcomes. This step is sometimes overlooked, and educational consultants are placed in the position of being an "advocate" of objectives. Their challenge is in helping staff develop meaningful objectives while seeing that they do not get "bogged down" or discouraged with detail.

Educational consultants might become involved in the development of unit orientation plans that build on the central orientation curriculum. They can offer recommendations on preliminary planning, format and content which will facilitate integration of unit and central orientation. Particular emphasis is placed upon using the principles of adult and self-directed learning for unit orientation as well as other staff development programs.

Organizing and Implementing

When a program has reached the combined stages of organization and implementation, nursing staff use educational consultants in the role of facilitators. The consultants can delineate available and appropriate learning resources, and assist the staff in the optimal utilization of selected resources. They can help the staff request budget money to purchase additional supplies, and prepare handouts or audio-visual aids for a program. They can also provide staff with guidelines and assistance in obtaining and operating audio-visual equipment or in scheduling an appropriate room.

Consultants have the responsibility of assisting staff in maintaining staff development records and obtaining CERPs. CE records are maintained by each staff member and are collected by the staff development representative to be placed in personnel files. These records are a requirement of the Joint Commission on Accreditation of Hospitals, but are especially useful by individuals for reference or resumés. Appropriate application forms are made available to nurses who wish to participate in the voluntary CERP program through the Washington State Nurses Association. Consultants may also become involved with the process of submitting appropriate unit educational programs for CERP credit.

An additional responsibility of educational consultants is to assist staff in obtaining and using budget money designated for programs outside of the hospital. Each unit is allocated a limited sum of money to be used as the unit desires. However, the staff may turn to their educational consultant to help them identify appropriate conferences or workshops according to learning needs and to distribute the funds as equally as possible.

The primary responsibility of educational consultants in the evaluation of a program involves assisting the staff in appraising the achievement of identified learning objectives. Since the major focus of staff development programs is on improved patient care, the staff is encouraged to observe changes in the delivery of health care that will demonstrate the effectiveness of a program. Consultants may also be involved in evaluation as related to professional job satisfaction and maintaining a climate conducive to continued learning.

Educational Consultant as Resource Person

At University Hospital Department of Nursing Services, the major responsibility for staff development is at the unit level. Each unit has a selected unit staff development representative and an assigned consultant from the staff development division. Educational consultants are one of many resource persons available to nursing units, but they have specific responsibilities in assisting staff in planning, organizing, implementing and evaluating staff development programs. At all times, they share responsibility with unit staff and other management level people to participate in the continual assessment of unit learning needs and to provide appropriate feedback.

Vicki C. Edwards, R.N., M.S.N.
Health Education Resources Coordinator II
Continuing Nursing Education
School of Nursing
University of Washington

THE ROLE OF THE NURSING UNIT STAFF DEVELOPMENT REPRESENTATIVE

The role of staff development representatives is multifaceted. They are responsible for seeking, from staff, areas of interest and coordinating programs with other disciplines to satisfy educational needs. They also act as liaisons between the staff development division and the nursing unit, are participants in implementing general hospital inservice programs, and develop innovative approaches to maintain staff involvement.

Staff development representatives are vital to the staff development system as they coordinate and focus the nursing staff's educational efforts. An example of an innovative approach occurred when I found that the staff was constantly teaching and exchanging new information with each other on an informal basis. When I asked the staff if they would like to present 15-minute mini-inservices once a week, the nurses were interested and enthusiastic. A sign-up sheet was initiated and I was presented with a wide variety of mini-inservices and full staff participation. The staff development representative is often called upon to provide the stimulus to get this type of program started.

The key to a successful unit staff development program is staff interest and participation. The staff is periodically asked to identify and list their clinical education needs and interests and those needs must then be met. To do this, a strong but flexible leadership is required. I have found that a democratic approach works well

The key to a successful unit CE program is staff interest and participation. The staff at University Hospital is periodically asked to identify and list their clinical education needs and interests.

and is essential when staff interest and involvement is high. But when staff involvement decreases, a somewhat autocratic approach becomes necessary to ensure that the staff's basic learning needs are met. Coordinators need to be sensitive to the staff's receptiveness to each approach and to adapt their approach accordingly. They also need to set learning priorities, to be open-minded about staff ideas, and to promote CE for the advancement of each individual's clinical knowledge.

Staff development representatives can become very frustrated due to the lack of time to coordinate programs, the high attrition rate of employees and the constant revision of educational materials. They can experience these frustrations with the system, but also derive a great deal of satisfaction from their role. I have found that CE decreases the staff's anxiety through increased knowledge and improved ability to solve problems in clinical settings. Staff members have grown professionally and demonstrate an increase in professional standards in their development of teaching booklets, nursing care modules, and the improvement in their delivery of primary nursing.

Gloria Craig, R.N.
NPIII
Medical-Surgical Unit
University Hospital

THE CLINICAL NURSE SPECIALIST *IS* A TEACHER

No, clinical nurse specialists at University Hospital have not resolved the role conflicts that have plagued our colleagues across the nation. Instead, we have learned to expect the conflicts that come with multiple role expectations and to live with the ambiguity. In a sense, we have come to appreciate the freedom that the ambiguity affords.

Expectations of the clinical nurse specialist job description are high but so is the freedom to be creative in how we approach the tasks at hand. Teaching is just one aspect of the role. It may well be the integrative element, however, of the service, educative, consultative and research components of the role.

As the job description is written, we are responsible for quality nursing care on our assigned units on a 24-hour basis. Priorities are placed in areas of assessment, intervention and evaluation of patient and/or family care problems, staff development and administrative maintenance projects. Within the organizational structure of the department, we are also actively involved in the participative management of nursing services and rotate through house coverage as senior nurse on duty on weekends, holidays and during vacation periods.

There currently are five clinical nurse specialists in the inpatient setting. Each approaches her role a little differently, according to her skills and the needs of the assigned units and the overall departmental demands. One of the five is responsible for developing and coordinating patient/family teaching programs within the department. A renal clinician, a cardiovascular clinician, a maternal and child clinician, and one for psychiatry complete the current picture. An oncology clinical nurse specialist and one with rehabilitation, neurology and/or gerontology expertise are being recruited, based on existing needs and projected patient care programs within the hospital.

Each clinician is assigned to be resource person for a number of units. For example, the patient/family teaching clinician also functions as resource person for the rehabilitation unit and for a general surgical unit. The cardiovascular clinician currently is chief resource for the critical care units as well as for a general medical unit and for a unit serving neurological, neurosurgical and cardiac surgery patients.

Teaching at the Unit Level

At the unit level, clinician teaching varies from informal role-modelling to formal classroom instruction. Classes may be held routinely or on a p.r.n. basis. The renal clinician, for example, has developed a structured dialysis educational program designed for nurses who have been employed for a minimum of six months on units utilizing dialysis. The program is five days in length and at least eight hours per day. It consists of theory and as much practical experience as is available in the hospital at the time. Visits to other dialysis centers in the area may be arranged. Learning modules are included to cover all aspects of renal disease and dialysis. Standards for transplantation, peritoneal dialysis and hemodialysis as developed by the American Association of Nephrology Nurses and Technicians are integrated into the program. Each participant is evaluated on completion. The renal clinician states as an expected outcome for her educational program that dialysis coverage can and will be provided on a 24-hour-a-day, seven-day-a-week basis, at University Hospital. She periodically reviews dialysis skills via a checklist and/or demonstration and updates staff skills to meet that goal.

A contract may be the mechanism for implementing teaching for a specific learning need. As psychiatric clinical nurse specialist, for instance, I have contracted with the nurse coordinators on the psychiatric units to develop a package seminar on group therapies. A four-session series will cover theory, methods and practical application in a milieu setting. All nursing staff will be expected to complete the series. Videotaping and role playing will be incorporated into sessions that demand active learner involvement. The expected outcome is to have all nursing staff demonstrate at least beginning level skills in group therapies and to be able to co-lead with more experienced staff. Some of the already expert group leaders will be developed as teachers and the liberal use of videotaping will make the series easily available to repeat as staffing changes necessitate.

Our 24-hour responsibility for staff development necessitates availability of learning experiences around the clock. Classes such as the critical care monitoring series are taught at times selected by the participants. That may mean that clinical nurse specialists are teaching classes on any or all three shifts.

Role Modelling

One of the most satisfying of our teaching roles is that of role model. Opportunities for direct patient care fluctuate tremendously, predicated on factors too numerous to mention here. One clinician attempts to carry one to two patients' families at a time with the goal of providing emotional support and using the process as a teaching experience for staff.

The consultative element of the clinical nurse specialist role is quite visible at University Hospital. Teaching implications are limitless. Patients are whole persons, not just fragmented systems. The complex nature of University Hospital patients, coupled with the highly specialized nursing units, demands that nursing consultation be readily available. The nurses on the obstetrics unit may need psychiatric nursing consultation on management of the high-risk obstetric patient with "acting out" behavior. Conversely, the psychiatry unit may require obstetric consultation for their postpartum schizophrenic patient. And the orthopedic unit may well seek help with the pregnant patient in traction. A patient with advanced Parkinson's Disease, requiring electroconvulsive therapy for her severe depression while on the neurology unit, precipitated for those nurses a crash course on management of the patient receiving shock therapy.

The administrative responsibilities assumed by the clinical nurse specialists function as a two-edged sword with many drawbacks and yet some redeeming benefits. While we all hope to be primarily clinicians, organizationally we are expected to assume a number of administratively oriented functions. On one hand, we acutely feel those responsibilities cutting through time available for clinical duties. On the other hand, the increased visability to units other than our own puts us in a position to be more familiar with the learning needs and learning environment of the entire hospital. Consultation is a teaching process. When the clinicians are functioning as senior nurses for the hospital, the opportunities for impromptu consultation are many. The increased familiarity cuts through many of the barriers that typically impede the consultative process.

In graduate school, I found myself bewildered by the frequent references to learning to live with ambiguity. After some time in the clinical nurse specialist role, I have felt the full impact of the stress associated with role ambiguity, and have survived. As we sort out our priorities in the vast job description in the face of the realities of the situation, we recognize that we cannot, in fact, do it all ourselves. Much of our job satisfaction must come from teaching others. And, in fact, the clinical nurse specialist *must* be a teacher!

Judy Folks, R.N., B.S.
Clinical Nurse Specialist
Department of Nursing Services
University Hospital

LEARNING RESOURCE CENTER

Learning is an internal, uniquely individualized process that is a continuous, integral part of nursing. As adult learners, we generally see ourselves as responsible, self-directed individuals. Self-directed learning is an established norm at University Hospital and is actively promoted by the nursing services department. Nurses assume responsibility for identifying individual or specific unit learning needs and seeking ways to meet those needs.

A recent study showed that all nurses surveyed participated in some form of continuous learning, but were more likely to participate in self-directed learning activities than in group oriented programs which were planned and managed by an instructor.[1] Such a study has not been done in this hospital, but an educational needs assessment was done in 1976 to collect information regarding the nursing staff's perception of their educational needs, types of resources needed, the best format for programs and the best method of making the resources available. Needs that were identified by the staff included: a place for educational programs; knowledge of available resources; staff involvement in educational programs; and improved resources to support orientation and continuing staff development needs. They also felt that increased priority should be placed on providing challenging educational opportunities to experienced staff. Staff expressed a willingness to seek and use learning resources within the hospital. Positive responses were given to the use of self-directed learning modules, audio-visual aids, resources in the nursing services library, a resource circulation system and a quiet place for study within the hospital.

Based on Self-Directed Education

As members of the nursing department and the staff development division, we believe that optimal professional and individual development towards self-actualization occurs when the individual actively participates in the learning process. We believe that it is our responsibility to promote participation of nursing staff in this process. It is also our responsibility to provide opportunities and resources to meet the expressed needs of the staff for self-directed learning.

It is the responsibility of the nursing department and the staff development division to provide opportunities and resources to meet the expressed needs of the staff for self-directed learning.

Our beliefs are reflected in one of our 1977–78 goals which is to continue development of resources for increased self-direction and individual staff responsibility for professional development. Plans to achieve this goal include:

- Development and organization of a nursing services LRC.

- Expansion of the nursing services library to include current and recommended "core" nursing references.
- Development of a learning resource locator to coincide with the nursing skills checklist format and to include types, location and availability of learning resources.

Development and Organization

The LRC is conceptualized as a physical facility in a centralized location which provides a variety of resources for self-directed learning and staff development programs. This concept is receiving particular attention in our division as a means of providing:

- Current professional books and journals which are catalogued and indexed.
- Recommended "core" nursing references.
- A resource file which includes resources for patient-family learning, staff development programs, professional development and standards.
- Self-directed critical care modules and related audio-visual aids.
- Self-directed learning resources which offer CERP for relicensure.
- A systematic method for circulation of resource material.
- A quiet area for independent study.
- Classroom space.
- Audio-visual equipment.

Further assessment of learning needs directly related to the concept of an LRC is necessary. A questionnaire is being developed which expands upon the 1976 educational needs assessment and will seek input regarding the purpose, projected use and desired resources for an LRC. Information which has already been gathered from the previous questionnaire and personal communications with nursing staff indicated a need to proceed with the concept. Coordination of the plans for development of the LRC became one of my primary responsibilities. After some initial thinking and discussion, I saw two major concurrent tasks ahead of me: 1) development, implementation and evaluation of an organization plan for an LRC, and 2) a written proposal which documented and justified the need for a physical facility for use as an LRC.

The organizational plan actually began with the needs assessment and conceptualization of an LRC. A review of literature was done during the early stages of planning, but was not particularly helpful in terms of developing a plan of action. However, a wealth of information was available in our health sciences library and other resource centers in the university system and other community hospitals.

Objectives

Initial objectives with activity and evaluation plans included: cataloging and indexing all resource material; designing a systematic method for circulation of resource material, and identifying and purchasing recommended "core" nursing and related health sciences references. The latter objective was developed after assessing our small library, nursing unit needs and reviewing two excellent articles on recommended books and journals.[2,3]

Other planning objectives involved the development of a resource file which would provide references for patient-family health care, classes, special projects or individual interests; development of independent study resources and facilities; and development of methods to promote utilization of nursing services library and the LRC in the future. Planning also incorporated a system whereby nursing staff could request additional learning resources and a system for assessment of the relevance and utilization of resources.

Implementation

To operationalize our concept of an LRC, we needed to think about a facility for library, study, classroom and office space. Lack of a physical facility, which would be centrally located and readily available to staff, quickly became an obvious problem in the implementation of the organizational plan for an LRC. The room which housed the existing nursing services library was frequently reserved for meetings and geographically removed from the nursing units.

During this time period, the hospital was undergoing a major phase of reconstruction. We learned that some hospital space in an ideal location would become available for negotiation. The timing was right to prepare a written proposal for presentation to hospital administration. Documentation of the need was relatively straightforward, stating the expressed needs of staff and documenting the unavailability of adequate resources. Justification presented for the concept of an LRC was twofold: 1) CE requirements of accrediting and other professional organizations, and 2) learning needs of nursing staff to meet role expectations of University Hospital.

JUSTIFICATION

I first turned to the Joint Commission on Accreditation of Hospitals as a source of national standards which greatly influence hospital operations. One of the standards established for nursing services states, "There shall be continuing training programs and educational opportunities for the development of nursing personnel."[4] The interpretation of this particular standard includes recommendations to make current professional books and journals available to nursing staff.

We were already in the process of updating and expanding the nursing services library, but the major concern was making the references available once they were obtained. The University's health sciences library generally meets the commission's standard for professional library services. However, I found that the interpretation of this standard specifically states, "There must be an adequate, readily available basic library that affords staff prompt access to current material."[5] The proposal documented the fact that the health sciences library does not provide quick accessibility to information which would facilitate problem solving and delivery of quality health care.

Optimal health care is not only the major concern of the Joint Commission on Accreditation of Hospitals, but also of the nursing profession. The quality of health care is contingent upon the knowledge and skills of the health care provider. Professional organizations are clearly indicating a belief that CE is requisite to maintaining and improving competency in practice. An example cited in the proposal was the *Position Statement on Nursing Licensure* from the National League for Nursing, which states: "The consumer should have assurance that the nurse is *currently* competent. A continuing education requirement for relicensure should be incorporated into state nurse practice acts."[6] The state of Washington appears to be moving toward mandatory CE for relicensure which will have an obvious impact on our nursing staff.

American Nurses' Association's *Standards for Continuing Education in Nursing* were used wherein it is stipulated that "The employer carries a responsibility to promote the continuing education of nursing personnel."[7] The Association's *Guidelines for Staff Development* were also used. These Guidelines encourage individual endeavors to identify learning needs and seek ways to meet these needs but also state that a staff development program must provide necessary resources and opportunities for self-directed learning.[8]

The concept of an LRC was also justified according to individual learning needs to meet role expectations at University Hospital. Continual emergence and application of new knowledge and technology is characteristic of a teaching and research hospital. Our nursing staff have an ongoing need for learning resources to maintain a level of skills and knowledge necessary for safe, competent patient care. The proposal also identified other characteristics of University Hospital which increase individual learning needs, such as: a nursing staff of primarily professional nurses, implementation of primary nursing and decentralized CE. Individual nurses are responsible and accountable for planning and implementing patient care, as well as individual and professional development.

REQUISITIONING SPACE

Given the identified needs of nursing staff, objectives and supporting rationale for the concept of an LRC, specific space was requested and a drawing of the proposed floor plan submitted. This plan fit into the space under consideration which was approximately 840 square feet and included all of our requests. Our plan would provide: room for a secretary at the entrance to monitor traffic and checkout procedures, a library with a small informal study area, a separate room for several study carrels and a classroom which would be approximately 350 square feet. This classroom had another entrance and could be divided by a folding partition to provide greater flexibility in use. The plan also provides two offices which would be approximately 88 square feet, which could accommodate four members of the staff development division. The facility would not be spaceous, but would help us over the major stumbling block in our planning.

In July 1977, the proposal had just been presented to the hospital administration by our acting director of nursing services, and the outcome pending. In the interim, negotiations were completed for the temporary use of a small room by the staff development division. We quickly decided to convert this room into a library with a reading and study area in order to operationalize that portion of our concept.

Benefits

An LRC has been presented as a method to provide a variety of resources to promote and facilitate self-directed learning and individual staff responsibility for professional development. Self-directed, one-to-one or group-directed activities can be utilized in implementing staff development programs. In addition, a more coordinated system of resources and programs can be provided to meet CE requirements of accrediting and professional organizations. Finally, the inherent flexibility and adaptability of an LRC would facilitate the process of keeping in step with the changing trends in health care.

REFERENCES

1. Clark, K. and Dickinson, G. "Self-Directed and Other-Directed Continuing Education: A Study of Nurses' Participation," *Journal of Continuing Education in Nursing* 7 (July-August 1976) p. 16–24.
2. Brandon, N. "Selected List of Books and Journals for the Small Medical Library," *Bulletin of Medical Library Association* 65:2 (April 1977) p. 191–215.
3. Interagency Council on Library Resources for Nursing. "Reference Sources for Nursing," *Nursing Outlook* 24 (May 1976) p. 317–322.
4. Joint Commission on Accreditation of Hospitals. "Accreditation Manual for Hospitals" (1976).
5. Ibid.
6. National League for Nursing. *Position Statement on Nursing Licensure* (1975).
7. American Nurses' Association Council on Continuing Education. *Standards for Continuing Education in Nursing* (1975).
8. American Nurses' Association. *Guidelines for Staff Development* (1975).

Vicki C. Edwards, R.N., M.S.N.
Health Education Resources Coordinator II
Continuing Nursing Education
School of Nursing
University of Washington

A MODEL FOR STAFF DEVELOPMENT

To be consistent with Nursing Services' philosophies concerning primary nursing, professional accountability and participative management, a model for CE was developed which includes self-directed learning opportunities for each nurse on the staff. (See Figure 2.) This model suggests a variety of learning experiences which nurses may pace to their own learning needs. Assistance to the nurse in identifying appropriate developmental programs is provided by either the nurse coordinator, staff development representative or educational consultant from the staff development division.

Individual Needs Assessment

After general orientation, developmental experiences at University Hospital are divided into two complementary and interdependent strands: a clinical strand and a management strand. New graduates (resident nurse practitioners or RNPs) focus first on identifying their own learning needs, a process facilitated by the nursing skills checklist. They can refer to the University Hospital Department of Nursing Management and Nursing Care Standards for a description of their expected role. The staff development division recognizes that, at this stage, the nurse's primary need is to develop clinical skills and confidence. The management strand is introduced through the management standards, and active participation of new staff is welcomed, but not emphasized at this time to allow the nurse time to get over the initial reality shock of the change from school to work.

Focus on Individual Growth

After about six to nine months of employment the staff nurse progresses to first level staff nurse (NPI). At this stage, developmental emphasis in the clinical strand is on promotion of individual growth through gaining additional confidence in nursing skills. The staff nurse is aided in this process through both unit-based and general inservice presentations. Each unit develops clinically-oriented educational materials specific to its patient population. Many units also require the arrhythmia analysis course at this point as a condition to advancement to NPII so the nurse may be in charge of the unit. In the management strand, nurses may participate in the leadership program or they may defer it until they become NPIIs. They may begin to take a more active role in unit management as a participating staff member and may decide to join and contribute to a nursing services' committee.

Experienced staff nurses (NPIIs) are clinically competent in basic skills and are ready to begin developing advanced expertise with self-instructional critical care modules. Since University Hospital is a tertiary, referral hospital for Washington, Idaho, Montana and Alaska, most of our patients can be defined as "critical care" in terms of their illnesses and the amount of nursing care they need. Expert clinicians in cardiovascular nursing, renal nursing, patient-family teaching, obstetrics and psychiatry are also utilized by nursing staff as consultants and role models. The need for resources for nursing staffs is constantly being assessed and as a result additional clinicians are presently being sought in the areas of oncology and neurology. As clinical experience develops, the nurse is able to begin assisting in the clinical orientation of new staff nurses. At this point, the leadership program which emphasizes interpersonal effectiveness, group process skills and defensible decision making is meaningful for the personal growth of many nurses.

Promoting Self-Growth

Promotion to assistant head nurse (NPIII) places the nurse in a formal managerial role. For example, the nurse is frequently in charge of the unit, plans new staff orientations and completes evaluations of individual staff members. To facilitate development of these and other managerial skills, a management seminar is offered three times a year. New NPIIIs are also provided with an individually planned orientation which acquaints them with other departments and their relations with nursing services. In the clinical strand, they have become expert clinicians who can be role models and teachers. In conjunction with the CE representative, they are able to identify and plan for meeting the educational needs of the nursing staff. They independently continue to identify and find opportunities to meet their own educational needs.

Expansion of Professional Experience

The final developmental level is open-ended and allows for continual growth of nurses as managers and clinical experts. Nurses participate more actively in nursing service goals in addition to individual unit goals. Upon appointment as NC, a preceptor experienced in management is appointed to assist the new NC in the refinement of managerial skills. Experienced NCs and clinicians provide their own CE by seeking outside or inhouse resources which meet their identified educational needs.

Advanced management seminars are presently being planned to provide continuing managerial education for this group. CE in clinical areas at this level is actively pursued through involvement in professional specialty organizations, attending advanced clinical seminars offered in the community and planning and presenting seminars through specialty organizations or through the Continuing Education Department of the University of Washington School of Nursing.

University Hospital's commitment to education and the philosophy of self-directed learning are two reasons why nurses find professional job satisfaction at this institution.

University Hospital's commitment to education, and the philosophy of self-directed learning are two reasons why nurses find professional job satisfaction at this institution.

Edna Zebelman, R.N., M.S.
Lecturer, Graduate Program in Nursing Administration
University of Washington

NURSING LEADERSHIP DEVELOPMENT PROGRAM

Nursing Services has planned two programs as a developmental series in the management strand for staff nurses. These are entitled Nursing Leadership Development Program (leadership) and Creative Management for Nursing Leaders (management). Both programs are held as a series of three all-day seminars.

Objectives

The leadership program is designed to fulfill a felt need to promote more independence among staff nurses practicing primary nursing. Bailey's definition of leadership as a set of actions which influence members of a group to move towards an identified goal is used as a conceptual framework for the program.[1] In this sense, all professional nurses at University Hospital should be prepared to assume a leadership role. To promote more confident and effective leaders, certain behaviors can be developed through a planned educational experience.

The leadership program is designed to develop basic leadership skills such as self-confidence and interpersonal effectiveness, assertiveness, visible professional accountability, group process skills and defensible decision making. The main focus of the program is on the self, as a leader of people. This program is open to all staff RNs with the approval of their NC. After participation in the program, it is hoped that learners will be able to:

- Increase their self-awareness.
- Employ techniques of open communication in daily practice and to facilitate communication among others.
- Express a growing sense of individual accountability in more extensive practice of primary nursing as evidenced by problem-oriented recording and nursing care plans.
- Use and share with others systematic problem-solving and decision-making techniques.
- Evaluate people and situations in a systematic fashion.

The self-development goal of this program necessitates active learning in which the learner participates in all phases of the learning process. Information in the form of lecturing or reading is incidental to the process through which the participant integrates concepts into professional practice. This goal is supported through the use of small group discussions, role playing and other situational learning experiences.

One problem with leadership has been the uncertainty with which some participants enter the program. They may be unsure about the concept of self-directed learning or even why they are in a leadership program since they define a "leader" as an NPIII or NC. Some have heard positive feedback from peers about the program, some have heard negative feedback and some attend because "my NC thought it would be good for me."

To help participants focus their learning needs, I recently designed a "planning tool for educational effectiveness" which functions as an educational contract. The tool asks the participants to:

- Prioritize their learning needs in terms of the course objectives.
- Plan for achieving their primary objectives.
- Identify behavioral changes they will try to make as a result of their participation.
- Describe in what ways these be-

havioral changes will affect their nursing care delivery.

The tool has been helpful in compelling participants to really scrutinize their reasons for attending the program and what they hope to accomplish as a result of their participation.

The final part of the tool states: "Hopefully this leadership program will give you some insight into yourself and some tools to better practice primary nursing. What do you plan to give in return to your fellow participants in this group?" I designed this question to emphasize learning as an active sharing process rather than the passive "sponge-like" process which some nurses have come to expect from a formal educational experience. As program coordinator, this tool has also given me helpful feedback. For example, accountability is often the last priority for many participants as they feel that they are already professionally accountable. This has led me to spend less time discussing accountability as a separate section and to integrate concepts and demonstration of accountability into discussions on other topics.

The most frequent top priority choices are open communication and problem-solving. Many participants feel some weakness in problem-solving skills and want to work to improve them. Poor communication with peers and other disciplines is a continual source of stress for many staff nurses. In response to feedback in this area, I recently added a session on management of personal stress which has been very helpful to participants.

Presentation Format

The leadership program is offered as a series of three all-day workshops. It has generally been presented on three consecutive Tuesdays as this appeared to be the best day for NCs to schedule participants to be off the units. The number of participants in any one series has ranged from eight to 14 with 11 or 12 seeming ideal. A tone of informality is set through a circular seating arrangement and having a coffee pot in the room. I also try to eliminate the typical classroom image by using the words ***program*** instead of ***class*** or ***course*** and ***coordinator*** instead of ***teacher.*** Another way of dispelling a formal atmosphere is to be as flexible as possible in allowing the group to go off on tangents for a while when they are having a heated discussion.

The first morning begins with an unfreezing, get-acquainted exercise called **first names, first impressions.**[2] The group then breaks into small groups to come up with a definition of leadership, the skills needed by a leader, which of those skills they feel proficient in and which they need to develop further, and finally in what ways they see themselves as leaders in their present roles. This discussion is frequently enlightening as the participants define a "leader" with typical head nurse behaviors. Leadership skills which the head nurse needs are identified as motivating others, conflict-resolution, assertiveness and good communication. We then discuss the leadership definition on which the program is based so that we all have the same orientation.

To further clarify the program goals, we discuss power as a positive force and that the program is designed to give them skills to potentiate their own power as nurses. The concept of **synergic power,** "The capacity of an individual or group to increase the satisfactions of all participants by intentionally generating increased energy and creativity, all of which is used to cocreate a more rewarding present and future,"[3] is used to diminish some negative connotations of the use of the word "power." The rest of the morning is spent discussing accountability, in terms of individual responsibility for professional practice and of identification of techniques to increase documentation of nurse accountability.

The afternoon of the first day is devoted to open communication and interpersonal effectiveness. I have tried a variety of experiences in this session, some of which were more or less successful than others. The success of many exercises depends to a great extent on the "mix" of participants. Some groups jump right in and enjoy participating and others need to go a little more slowly until they feel more secure in the situation. The most successful exercises have been the Johari Window using Johnson's **Friendship Relations Survey,**[4] **Three-minute Sharing,**[5] and using some role-playing situations which illustrate assertiveness principles.

The morning of the second day is spent in developing group process skills. This session is led by Barbara Larson, an evening supervisor who has had extensive experience in group process work. Barbara uses an experience-reflection model of instruction and role play to give participants opportunities to experience unfamiliar group roles and to practice group roles which they wish to develop in themselves.

The Claus-Bailey Model for Systematic Problem Solving is introduced during the afternoon of the second day.[6] Emphasis is placed on identifying the *true* cause of a problem as one of the first steps in the decision-making process. Each group chooses a problem to "work through the model" so that the process is meaningful for it. This project is continued through the morning of the third day. These two sessions receive mixed reviews. Many participants are very excited by and interested in systematic decision making while a few feel the process is too long and drawn out.

The final afternoon is spent winding up. Some free time is given to the group to use as it wishes. This time may be used to practice group process skills, to review parts of the decision-making process or to engage in exercises which focus on sharing and trust.

A recent addition to the program has been a session on personal management of stress. Participants share with each other sources of work-related stress and their means of coping with it. Group members are very supportive of each other and identify with each other's feelings.

To end the program with positive feelings, I use an exercise called **the gift of happiness: experiencing posi-**

tive feedback.[7] Each participant writes personalized, positive feedback notes to five randomly assigned group members. This is a very happy experience which points out how infrequently we receive positive feedback from our peers. Participants say they will save their messages to read as an "upper" on a particularly "down" day.

Participant Evaluation

On the first day of the program, all participants receive three copies of an evaluation worksheet which they in turn give to three coworkers, either peer, subordinate or superior. The questions of the worksheet are phrased to provide descriptive rather than evaluative comments on the participants' behaviors in relation to the major objectives of the program. At the end of the program, participants collect these worksheets and in turn write a self-evaluation of their learning as a result of the program.

Program Evaluation and Evolution

The program is evaluated both through verbal feedback and with a standard nursing services course evaluation questionnaire. Both of these methods have given me feedback which I have then used to make meaningful changes. One thing I have learned through experience is not to always make changes as a result of one group's feedback. For example, due to the individual characteristics of each group, an exercise which falls flat with one group will be very successful with the next group. Feedback on the program and on me as the coordinator is honest and thoughtful. It has been very helpful in tailoring the program to the changing needs of the nurses in this hospital.

The leadership program has now been offered 13 times over a two-year period. Although it has continually evolved to meet changing needs, it is now time for a more complete restructuring of the program. I have found that staff nurses do not understand the Nursing Services organization process and the way in which they can contribute to the system. Although this is covered in general orientation, nurses do not seem to "hear" it as they have other priorities at that time. A brief history of reorganization would be appropriate in the program as a means of illustrating nursing's power for change. Other program changes might include less emphasis on accountability as a separate topic and less time spent on the decision-making model.

I feel that the program has contributed significantly to staff nurses by helping them to learn and practice leadership skills which in turn encourages them to be more confident and effective primary nurses.

The leadership program at University Hospital has contributed significantly to staff nurses by helping them to learn and practice leadership skills which in turn encourages them to be more confident and effective primary nurses.

REFERENCES

1. Bailey, J. T. and Claus, K. E. *Decision Making for Nurses: Tools for Change* St. Louis: (C. V. Mosby, 1975).
2. Jones, J. E. in Pfeiffer, J. W. and Jones, J. E., eds. *A Handbook of Structured Experiences for Human Relations Training* Vol. II (Iowa City: University Associates Publishers and Consultants 1972) p. 88–90.
3. Craig, H. H. and Craig, M. *Synergic Power: Beyond Domination and Permissiveness* (Berkeley, Calif.: Proactive Press 1973) p. 62.
4. Johnson, D. W. Reaching Out: *Interpersonal Effectiveness and Self-Actualization* (Englewood Cliffs, N.J.: Prentice-Hall 1972) p. 21–25.
5. Stewart, J. and D'Angelo, G. *Together: Communicating Interpersonally* (Reading, Mass.: Addison-Wesley 1975.
6. Bailey and Claus, Decision Making for Nurses.
7. Keyworth, D., Pfeiffer, J. W. and Jones, J. E., eds. *A Handbook of Structured Experiences for Human Relations Training* Vol. IV (Iowa City: University Associates Publishers and Consultants 1973) p. 15–17.

Edna Zebelman, R.N., M.S.
Lecturer, Graduate Program in Nursing Administration
University of Washington

SELF-EVALUATION OF LEARNING IN THE LEADERSHIP PROGRAM

The leadership program in which I recently participated fell at an opportune time for my personal growth. I feel particularly "teachable" in matters related to leadership, since I intend to apply shortly for a leadership position in my nursing unit. The opportunity to learn, review and practice the concepts presented in the course has resulted in amazing attitudinal changes within me. More behavioral changes should result as I further assimilate the knowledge and become more comfortable with these ideas.

During the course, I was aware of bolstering of my self-confidence. I feel that the contributing causes were in part: hearing the reactions of previous strangers to me; feeling a mutual sharing of ideas with nurses from various units; and seeing the attentiveness with which the group members responded to each other.

I have usually been seen by myself and others as an assertive person, but know that I have tendencies toward over-aggressiveness. The opportunity to deal with characteristics of assertiveness made me greatly aware of examples in which I was assertive, helped me to use assertion appropriately, and helped me stop short of the "aggressive stage" in some situations. Examples seen by others were:

- When a physician told me to do a procedure that was his responsibility, I discussed the situation with him to explain why I objected to the order.
- In a joint staff meeting, I stated my feelings of displeasure with the attitudes of OR nurses when they are asked to help with C-sections.
- I explained to a physician the nurse's side of the question of whether to do a D&C in the DR or the OR.

The incidents I can recall are numerous, which pleases me. I have also been assertive in instances outside the hospital, such as insisting on several repairs in my apartment that the manager has put off for months, and discussing with my roommate the frustration I feel when she borrows things without asking me.

Having always been one who is very quick to speak up and answer a question, and prone to inappropriate interruptions of others, the course reminded me that I had become slack in my intentions to improve. My incentive was built-up, so I am now concentrating on reducing this tendency, and the results have been obvious to myself and peers.

I have made efforts to participate in informal peer review by asking and offering thoughts on general behavioral characteristics and on specific situations. Along with this, I have made certain to show others that I appreciate and respect their opinions.

Problem solving has always been something I enjoy and feel challenged by, so I was fascinated by the Claus-Bailey method of problem solving which we studied and practiced.[1] In several instances, I have been able to work through problems more effectively and logically by giving thought to specific steps in the solution. A peer described that I am able to "exhibit a little more patience to ascertain the 'feel' of a situation and give a more gentle response," rather than to just "jump in with both feet."

The course enlightened me in many aspects of professional nursing. I joined the CERP program after learning its benefits, have vowed to become more active in Washington State Nurses Association, and plan to learn more about the functions and actions of Nursing Services. I have been more attentive in my care plans and charting, and have been working as primary nurse for a complicated patient. I see the course as having been a major step in the development of what I want to be in nursing.

REFERENCE

1. Bailey, J. T. and Claus, K. E. *Decision Making for Nurses: Tools for Change* (St. Louis: C. V. Mosby 1976).

Sally Avenson, R.N., B.S.
NPIII
Obstetrics Unit
University Hospital

CREATIVE MANAGEMENT FOR NURSING LEADERS

Creative Management for Nursing Leaders is a series of three all-day seminars offered three times a year. It is open to newly appointed NPIIIs, who have not yet had a chance to attend, new NCs, and NCs who have identified a need to refresh their knowledge of management theories and techniques. Efforts are made to ensure that new NPIIIs and NCs attend as soon as possible after their appointment.

This seminar has been developed for managers at the nursing unit level and is designed to assist these managers in identifying and employing skills which will maximize each unit's potential for quality nursing care delivery as well as professional satisfaction for the staff and the manager.

To clarify the distinction between leadership and management we cite

Hersey's and Blanchard's concept that leadership is broader than management.[1] A leader tries to impact the behavior of an individual or group for a given specific reason. The reason a manager tries to impact the behavior of an individual group is for the purpose of achieving *organizational* goals. We also believe that the most important managerial skill is the ability to work *through* people rather than *for* them. Nurse managers need to develop skills which will enable them to involve the entire nursing staff in the total management of the unit.

Central Objectives

We realize that a three-day seminar can only begin to touch the surface of modern management theory. To stimulate self-directed learning in this area, we provide an extensive syllabus with: specific learning objectives for each topic; one assigned reading for each topic from either the textbook or relevant journals; reprints of assigned journal readings; a textbook;[2] and additional bibliographical references on each topic.

At the conclusion of this seminar, it is anticipated that each participant will be able to:

- Recognize the responsibilities of the management role on the nursing unit and in the total health care organization.
- Assist the nursing staff in defining goals for the improvement of nursing care.
- Plan, implement and assess unit orientation and continuing education programs for nursing staff.
- Devise a staffing pattern balancing patient activity needs, employee needs and the unique needs of each unit.
- Apply principles of motivation theory and human behavior in effecting change.
- Apply principles of effective communication in her interactions with others in the health care setting.
- Utilize interviewing and counseling skills in the development of nursing staff.
- Plan, in conjunction with the nursing staff, for meaningful and systematic performance reviews.
- Design an organizational plan to facilitate the efficient functioning of the nursing unit.
- Apply the philosophy of nursing services to her activities and goals.
- Plan and evaluate a program for her own self-development in the leadership role.
- Create a positive climate for the assumption of individual professional accountability by the nursing staff.

Presentation Format

Individual sessions in the management seminar are led by a variety of experts from Nursing Services and the community. The seminar is designed to include the classic management steps of **planning, organizing, implementing** and **evaluating.**

The first day is devoted to **planning.** Topics include the management process, the philosophy of participative management, management by objectives, nurse-nurse contracting and change theory. Ample time is given to participants to practice writing and to receive feedback on management objectives.

Organizing is the focus of the morning of the second day. A panel presentation on staffing discusses contractual staffing, patient classification, planning and daily problem solving necessary to meet total hospital needs, and the concept of negotiated workload.[3,4] Time management and delegation are discussed in another session. The final session of the morning is a role-playing experience utilizing a continuum of leadership styles to examine the effects of each style on the leader and the group.

Implementing is discussed in the afternoon. The orientation coordinator discusses planning for staff development and unit orientation. The second session deals with motivation theories and how to use these theories on the nursing unit. The final session of the day covers identifying and dealing with group problems such as apathy, inadequate decision making and discord. Implementing is continued on the third day with discussion on identifying and intervening to cope with work-related stress among staff. The final implementing session is an experimental learning exercise in conflict resolution.

The **evaluating** segment of the seminar is composed of an experiential learning exercise on performance evaluations and a discussion of quality assurance programs, especially nursing audit and peer review.

Participant Evaluation

Participants are evaluated by means of a MBO worksheet. All participants write two management objectives for their unit and plan for their implementation and evaluation. They are encouraged to incorporate concepts discussed during the seminar into their plan.

In addition, the most recent (April 1977) management seminar participants will be evaluated with a pre/post competencies form which attempts to measure perceived changes in management skills competencies. The three-month post-test will be sent out next month.

Seminar Evaluation

The seminar presentations are evaluated by participants using a worksheet which lists each topic and its presentor. The participant receives this form on the first day and is encouraged to write a comment or evaluation on each topic as soon as possible after its presentation. Completed forms are circulated to all presentors who then use feedback to improve their presentations for the next time.

This feedback has also been used to add or delete topics from the seminar. Recent feedback on a session on delegation indicated a need to include delegation in the new, broader topic of time management. We also incorporated a separate session on principles of interviewing into performance evaluations.

As in the leadership program, participant feedback is an important source of information for the continual refinement of the management seminar. Another source of change is the CE of each of the presentors. In these and other ways, the seminar continually evolves to meet the current needs of nurse-managers at University Hospital.

REFERENCES

1. Hersey P. and Blanchard, K. H. *Management of Organizational Behavior: Utilizing Human Resources* 3rd Ed. (Englewood Cliffs, N.J.: Prentice-Hall 1977) p. 4.
2. Stevens, B. J. *The Nurse as Executive* (Wakefield, Mass.: Contemporary Publishing 1975).
3. Pardee, G. "Classifying Patients to Predict Staff Requirements," *American Journal of Nursing* 68:3 (1968) p. 517–520.
4. Fine, R. B. "Controlling Nurses' Workload," *American Journal of Nursing* 74:12 (1974) p. 2206–7.

Edna Zebelman, R.N., M.S.
Lecturer, Graduate Program in Nursing Administration
University of Washington

MANAGEMENT SEMINAR PRINCIPLES PUT INTO PRACTICE

I am in a new management role at University Hospital as assistant head nurse in charge of the evening shift of a clinical research unit. After a month in the position I listed the following personal goals:

- To learn to manage time.
- To be an effective participant in peer evaluation.
- To decide what style of leadership is right for me.
- To learn to effectively orient new staff.
- To find ways to help nurses become more responsible for themselves.
- To help improve job satisfaction.

I needed help with organizing and implementing the above goals, so I requested that I attend the three-day management seminar.

The objective on which I concentrated was learning to manage my time more effectively. In the class, we were given a list of ten reasons why one wasted time. Five definitely applied to me: lack of priority setting, not taking time to organize, attempting too much, continually coordinating meetings to make decisions and saying "yes" too often. I now try to set priorities with a list of things to do, and the list is limited. I make independent decisions without group meetings when it is appropriate and have learned to say "no" before I am overwhelmed. I find myself working with time instead of working against it.

Self-Evaluation

Evaluation was a word that scared me. How could I be more effective in the evaluation process? In class we reviewed ways of evaluating, reasons for evaluating, and what to evaluate. I enjoyed the discussions of feelings about evaluating staff, finding that other new management people were as uneasy as I, while those that had done many evaluations were more comfortable. Two ideas reinforced in class were that evaluation is done not only to tell what staff nurses are doing wrong but also what they are doing right, and that evaluations enhance staff development throughout the process of goal setting, interviewing and ongoing followup. I try to evaluate, in terms of event language, "what happened?" I try to make expectations known to staff prior to evaluation, and I am beginning to record followup observations, to write contracts with staff and to keep current anecdotal notes.

I hoped in taking the class to learn and experience through role play, different types of nursing leadership styles. Through role-playing I found that what I thought was my democratic way of leading was actually a laissez faire style. I set a new goal for myself to lead in a fashion of fostering more independence in nurses, encouraging two-way communication and developing a participatory group.

With half of the evening staff possibly leaving in several months, orienting many new staff is a problem to be faced! Information for orienting staff is in three different areas of the unit, and even more information is in the heads of experienced staff. The need for forming orientation guidelines for new staff is urgent. Suggestions for the form, format, principles and content of orientation guidelines were introduced in the management class. Writing orientation guidelines is a nursing unit goal for 1978. I hope to contribute to the achievement of this goal by sharing information from the management seminar.

Promoting Accountability

I am interested in promoting professional accountability among nurses. Two potential ways of promoting accountability on our unit are nursing audit and contractual staffing. Methods introduced for nursing audit during the seminar were retrospective chart review and concurrent care monitoring. As a result of a retrospective chart audit, we identified the need for and developed nursing standards for the care of ophthalmology and oral surgery patients. We are now in the process of planning a concurrent care monitoring audit using these standards as a basis.

Staffing has become a problem on our unit because of the excessive amount of management time required to make out the monthly schedule. This process is further complicated by the large number of specific days for work and off-duty being requested by staff. This traditional method of scheduling involves almost no effort on the part of staff nurses and they are happy as long as their requests are met. The person making out the schedule is not very happy though, as she tries to fulfill everyone's requests. Contractual staffing promotes nurses' accountability by making them responsible for bidding for a position and exchanging with their peers for any necessary days off.

Meeting Goals

Since the listing of my goals as a new management person, I have found that they correlate directly with our unit goals. The discussions with other management persons, the talks given by resource people, the volunteering of resource people as an ongoing pool of knowledge has benefited me in my own goals as well as our unit's goals. The fantastic part of the management class for me has been using the knowledge I gained in implementing new plans, evaluating these plans and seeing that setting goals and making plans does help in my new managerial role.

Elaine Reams, R.N., B.S.
NPIII
University Hospital

NURSING SKILLS DEVELOPMENT WORKSHEET

It was with a certain amount of misgiving that the staff development division decided to develop the nursing skills development worksheet as a tool for the phantom unit orientation. These misgivings were founded on an inherent dislike of the checklist method of orientation and a wish to avoid overemphasis on the importance of technical skills by the orientees and the staff serving as orientors.

The misgivings were overcome by facing the reality that new nurses, especially new graduates, feel a need to become proficient in technical skills and often have to overcome this need before they can become fully involved in the nontechnical aspects of their roles. We further justified our misgivings by determining that the skills worksheet would be something more than the usual checklist. In addition to technical skills, the worksheet includes communications, psychosocial skills, philosophy of nursing, support services, leadership skills and learning resources for all of the items listed.

Purpose

The stated purpose of the worksheet addressed to the learners is to:

- Provide a tool for assessment and documentation of the present level of skill in applying nursing theory to patient care and performing various nursing care procedures.
- Document the level of skill nurses would like to attain during the first three to four months of employment at University Hospital.
- Assist in prioritizing learning and professional developmental needs.
- Inform nurses of resources available to assist in meeting these needs.
- Provide a tool for documentation of the attainment of the expected level of skill development.
- Provide data that can serve as a basis for self-evaluation and goal setting.
- Provide data that can be used by nurses and NCs for evaluation of developmental progress and discussion of goals and plans.

Format

Some of the ideas for format were taken from a self-directed orientation form used by one of the private industries in the area. The first pages of the worksheet contain the purpose, instructions and keys for documenting skill level and identifying learning resources.

In the body of the worksheet, the first column lists the skills grouped under appropriate headings. The next column asks for an assessment of present skill level with a one (inexperienced) to four (expert) ranking. The third column asks for a determination of the skill level the orientee would like to reach during the first three to four months of employment. Next is a request to prioritize the achievement of the skills on a one (highest priority) to five (lowest priority) ranking. Learning resources are identified in the fifth column and the last column is for documenation of the date achieved.

Content Selection

Selection of content was difficult. When one considers all the skills necessary for nurses working in all areas of the hospital, the list could be endless. Selection was focused on making the worksheet general to the medical-surgical nursing units. The selection process was aided by use of data from the needs assessment. As a part of that assessment, the NCs were asked to specify skills in which they expected their staff to be proficient and those they expected of float nurses assigned to their units.

Future Plans

There have not been any nurses assigned to the phantom unit since completion of the worksheet, so its usefulness for this type of orientation has not been assessed. At the present time, it is being tried for use by all orientees assigned to the medical-surgical nursing units. If the tool proves useful, unit nursing staffs will be given the option of adding a section on "unit specific" skills for each individual nursing unit.

Thelma Mackey, R.N., M.S.N.
Orientation Coordinator
Division of Staff Development
University Hospital

PHANTOM UNIT

Definition and Purpose

The phantom unit is a method of providing orientation for newly employed RNs who are not assigned to a specific nursing unit at the time of their employment. Each nurse is assigned to a nursing unit for orientation on a weekly rotating schedule. The phantom unit concept was conceived as a part of the Nursing Services reorganization plan to create a system which would:

- Provide Nursing Services with a pool of nurses who could be assigned to the nursing units as staff positions were vacated.

- Bridge the time gap between the termination of nurses and the time at which their replacements would become fully functioning staff members.
- Provide newly employed nurses with a planned orientation which would meet their particular needs.
- Decrease the large amount of time spent in one to one orientation of new staff by unit nursing staff.

The basic orientation plan and timetable of approximately six weeks is designed to prepare the newly graduated nurse to assume a RNP role on a general medical or surgical nursing unit. There is also planned flexibility to allow for individual differences, past experience and anticipated assignment to a specialized nursing unit. If a staff vacancy occurs on a nursing unit to which an orientee wishes to be assigned on a permanent basis, the orientee may be transferred before completion of the phantom unit orientation. The assigned person on that unit responsible for orientation is informed of the orientee's progress and experiences so that the two of them can plan to meet the remaining orientation needs. If an opening on a nursing unit of choice has not occurred when the phantom unit orientation is completed, the nurse will be given a temporary assignment.

Responsibility for the Phantom Unit

The staff development division has responsibility for the phantom unit with the orientation coordinator having primary responsibility for planning and coordination of the unit. Written plans include an overview or explanation of the phantom unit, goals, objectives, learning resources, evaluation forms and nursing skills worksheet. Each new phantom unit nurse meets with the staff development preceptor for an initial planning session and at regular times thereafter for assessment of progress and any changes in planning that may be needed.

Who Becomes a Phantom Nurse?

Over the past three years, the number of nurses in the phantom unit at any time has varied from none to eight. The following are some examples of situations in which orientees have been placed in the phantom unit:

- The director of nurses hires in advance for predicted peak times of staff turnover and there are not as many terminations as anticipated.
- Occasionally, the director of nurses places nurses in the phantom unit who exhibit a great deal of uncertainty about the type of nursing unit to which they would like to be assigned.
- As a part of the preparation for the opening of a new nursing unit, a number of newly hired nurses and nurses requesting transfer to the new unit became phantom unit nurses prior to the opening of the unit. These nurses can then have opportunities to care for the types of patients which will be on the new units.

Future Plans

Plans for the future are that all newly employed RNs will be oriented by the phantom unit method. This plan is dependent to some extent on budget approval. With the recent addition of personnel to the staff development division and assignment of individuals in the division as resource persons to the individual nursing units, responsibility for the phantom unit orientation will become more diversified. It is also planned that the staff development staff will increase their time and responsibility for unit orientation of the phantom unit nurses. This will relieve nursing unit staffs of some of the burden of orientation of new staff nurses.

Further development of existing written materials and development of self-learning modules in certain areas is currently being done. This will result in an orientation guide which will promote self-directed learning by the orientee. The orientation guide may also serve as a model for nursing unit staff who wish to develop orientation guides specific to the patient population of the unit.

Evaluation

There has not at this time been any formalized evaluation of the phantom unit concept. One of the obvious questions that arises when considering full implementation is cost. Current budgetary allocations allow for a two week time span between hiring of new employees and termination of the staff they are replacing. It is, of course, highly unrealistic to expect an experienced nurse, much less a new graduate, to become a fully functioning staff member in two weeks.

Improved patient care and decreased staff turnover could provide some justification for increased cost. Perhaps the answer for the future for our phantom unit and internship programs in other institutions lies in a three-way acceptance of the burden by the institutions, schools of nursing and the employees themselves.

Two problems identified by phantom unit nurses have been a feeling of not really "belonging" anywhere, and some staff on the nursing of not really "belonging" anywhere, and some staff on the nursphantom unit nurses. The first problem was partly overcome at times by scheduling weekly informal lunch meetings of nurses in the phantom unit. With full implementation of the concept the nurses may not feel as isolated as their group will be larger and they will meet as a group regularly for educational purposes and problem solving. The second problem is seen as a need for staff development resource people to meet with unit staff to provide them with the needed information and to answer questions. This problem should also decrease as CE resource people become more actively involved in orientation of the phantom unit nurses at the unit level.

Informal contact with phantom unit nurses following their orientation and with nursing unit staff suggests that the former phantom unit nurses may be more satisfied with their jobs than those nurses who did not have this experience. They have had an opportunity to observe the various nursing units and be observed by the unit staffs. In this way, the nurse can make a more informed choice about the nursing unit to which she would like to be assigned, and the unit NCs can make a more informed decision about accepting the nurses as additions to their staff. At one time, there were five phantom unit nurses requesting placement on the neonatal ICU. Since there were no openings and none anticipated soon, all five selected, and were selected by, other nursing units. The five were contacted ten months later and told they could request transfer to the neonatal unit. All stated that they preferred to remain where they were.

During the past year, ten nurses were oriented in the phantom unit with most of them beginning employment a full year ago. The usual turnover rate here is around 50 percent. Eight of the ten are still employed here and three have been observed to be active in Nursing Service committees as representatives of their nursing units.

Need for Similar Internship Programs

I believe that our phantom unit and similar internship programs in other institutions are very much needed, especially for orientation of the new graduates. Research illustrates dramatically the problems encountered by nurses in their transition from school to work settings.[1] A phantom unit type of orientation would not solve all of the problems but it should help by providing more structure and counseling during the initial stages of the adjustment from school to work.

REFERENCE

1. Kramer, M. *Reality Shock: Why Nurses Leave Nursing* (St. Louis: C. V. Mosby Co. 1974).

Thelma Mackey, R.N., M.S.N.
Orientation Coordinator
Division for Staff Development
University Hospital

PHANTOM UNIT: TWO PARTICIPANTS' VIEWPOINTS

Our initial reaction to University Hospital's phantom unit was one of amusement and curiosity. What was it? And why were we being introduced to such an elusive unit for our six-week orientation? Now, after four weeks on the unit, we

feel we were incredibly lucky and/or intelligent to have chosen it over a more specific unit. We are both new graduates and felt we could use more clinical expertise in many areas before we settled into the procedures that are routine to any individual unit. Neither of us preferred one area of nursing over another; in fact, we shared the belief that a broader experience in our initial weeks of orientation would best suit our needs. The phantom unit was suggested to us as a way of entering the system and providing an opportunity to observe the various units and become involved with the differing types of nursing and approaches to patient care.

As the days progressed, it became clear that we had made the right decision by joining the phantom unit, but for reasons that were only then becoming apparent.

Greater Flexibility

We rotated on a weekly basis to each unit and oriented to each, taking time to involve ourselves in patient care, develop nursing skills, and observe the structure and philosophy of the staff. We learned many more varied skills than would have been possible in six weeks if assigned to one area. By the second or third week, we became adept at searching out resources on each unit, e.g., the guidelines of care, patient teaching tools, reference books and bulletin boards posting inservices for continuing education. Because of our exposure to many units and the flexibility of skills this gave us, we felt more creative in our solutions to problems. An example of a patient with cancer on a medical floor needing more information about his daily blood count following a course of chemotherapy illustrates this point. On another unit where leukemia patients are followed, the nurses provide each patient with a simple flow sheet on which to chart daily lab results. No one had thought of this simple solution, but having seen its success on another unit prompted us to try it.

With this flexibility we saw our confidence and competence begin to develop. We also felt that the various experiences provided us more of an opportunity to enlarge on our own nursing styles, as we had not yet identified ourselves with one particular unit. Having observed how assorted nurses function on different units, we began to adapt our own individual methods of operation. For instance, one of us has found that she likes to make rounds on her patients directly following report, to introduce herself, bring linen, set up baths and corroborate the information obtained in report. Then she can check medications and take care of whatever else has come up, before the day gets into full swing.

The same process goes for treatments as well as routines—our criteria for action are synthesized and polished from many different sources. Furthermore, the theory emphasized so hard and for so long in nursing school doesn't quickly leave us—combining working on the units and meeting once or twice a week to talk over the program and to do independent study allows a good balance between academia and the realities (reality shock?) of working.

More In-depth Approach

With this broader, more in-depth approach to the units, we became aware of ourselves as contributors and resources on other units even in the midst of our orientation period. Because we could compare how things such as primary nursing and problem-oriented charting are done on the various floors, we could widen our circle of acquaintances. We feel that if everyone rotated as we did, we would not think of a unit as "the ophthalmology floor, I wonder what they do there?" but rather as "that's D and B's floor—I bet they'd know what we could do with Mr. Z." Resources become more apparent and, hence, better used.

Disadvantages Can Be Made to Work

There are disadvantages to joining the phantom unit, but some of these could be made to work for us. True, we don't feel as though we belong anywhere, and we lose the sense of responsibility that new graduates should develop as they make the transition from the role of student to that of RN. Many staff perceived our tentativeness as a characteristic associated with floating nurses. We were frequently perceived as orientees to the float pool, rather than as potential team members. Consequently, we found that the units were less inclined to involve us in the unit. As a result, we became more assertive, trying to publicize what a phantom is, to explain the distinction between a phantom and a float, and to be more aggressive in asking to watch and to do the various procedures on the floor. It's great to be able to determine your own learning needs and speeds, and to develop the habit of asking questions at every opportunity.

A final consideration is that of placement. Ideally, we should have a definite area in mind at the end of the six-week period. Because the phantom unit also serves as a holding unit, positions available before the completion of the orientation may require immediate placement of an interested phantom. Hence, the phantom unit experience might end prematurely.

The phantom unit has succeeded, for us, in promoting job satisfaction, increasing our competence and feelings of self-confidence, and making us more aware of the channels of communication and the structure of the health care system here. To aid in the effectiveness of this program, we would suggest that staff become better informed, either by orientation preceptors or the orientees themselves, of the nature and expectations of the phantom unit.

Carly Searles, R.N., B.S.N.
Staff Nurse
Obstetrics Unit

Kathleen Sullivan, R.N., B.S.N.
Staff Nurse
Surgical Unit
University Hospital

PLANNING A CENTRAL EDUCATION OFFERING: A PARTICIPATIVE APPROACH

Staff participative planning, as used by our staff development division, promotes support and involvement of staff at the unit level in a program from the planning stage to delivery date. With participative planning, staff programs focus on the needs of the personnel on nursing units rather then administrative needs.

Planning a Legalities Program

The legalities and liabilities workshop for nurses, which our staff presented this year, would be an example of participative planning.

When I joined the staff development division, the idea for a legalities conference had been circulating in the department for about a year. I was asked to pursue the idea.

My first priority was to ask the nursing staff members if the program was needed. I sent a letter to all unit staff development representatives and other personnel that might be interested in a legality conference. They were asked to attend a meeting to discuss the possibility of presenting a conference.

At the end of the first meeting the committee had decided there was a definite need for some type of legal program. We also discussed possible subject matter, speakers, format and presentation dates.

The planning committee met formally seven times over the next three months. Our meetings were interspersed by unit staff meetings. This allowed the staff development representatives to keep their staffs informed on the progress of the conference, and to solicit new ideas. Minutes of each meeting and personal contact kept the staff development representatives that could not attend the meetings informed of our progress.

The workshop was based on questions solicited from each nursing unit to determine common concerns on legal responsibilities. The staff development representatives were responsible for compiling questions from their individual units. I was responsible for correspondence with speakers, room arrangements, videotaping and coordinating the planning committee. Other committee members were active in preparing a bibliography list and publicity. The committee was also used for problem solving when speakers decided they would not be able to participate, when rooms were suddenly not available on the workshop date, and when back ordered videotaping equipment did not arrive on time.

A Successful Plan

Growing interest in the workshop was evident as the presentation date grew closer. The staff was talking about the conference. They were arranging their work schedules so they could attend. Those that could not attend were making arrangements for viewing the videotapes of the program.

The workshop was planned for nursing staff members, by staff members. It was based on information the staff requested.

Based on the high attendance at the program, feedback from the staff, requests for viewing the videotapes and future programs, our planning was a success.

Chris Moss, R.N.
Former Instructor
Division of Staff Development
University Hospital

EPILOGUE, APRIL 1982

Since the initial series of articles were written for *Nursing Administration Quarterly*, a number of changes have occurred in the Department of Nursing Staff Development at University Hospital. Some have occurred because of the inevitable change that takes place when "new blood" enters the organization, bringing with it new approaches, interests and skills. Some have occurred through development and expansion of already existing concepts, and some have occurred because of the availability of new facilities and equipment. I would like to share briefly some of the most significant changes so that you have a current "on-the-scene" view.

With the support of our current nursing administrator, Irma Goertzen, R.N., F.A.A.N., and our hospital administrator, Rob Muilenburg, the space we desired for the Learning Resource Center was secured, and the Learning Resource Center has been completed. It includes a library for storage of books, journals, self-directed learning modules and audio-visual materials; a classroom that can be divided into two smaller classrooms, a small skills laboratory facility in one of the classrooms, space for equipment storage and office space.

Another change has been the addition of an educational strand to the already existing clinical and leadership curriculum strands in the Model for Staff Development. (See Figure 3.) This is consistent with the development of a career ladder within our organization that includes an educational tract. It is also consistent with our goal to assist individuals in the organization to be self-directed and accountable for their own professional development. We feel that many staff are not prepared with the knowledge, skill or experience necessary to assume this responsibility, and that we have an obligation to assist them to become competent in the practice of adult learning. We begin this process on the first day of orientation where staff complete and discuss the "Learning Styles Inventory."[1] This assists them to analyze their own preferred style of learning and to be intentional in considering the transition from a teacher, classroom and textbook style of learning to a more active self-directed style of learning.[2] They gain practice during the orientation period in analyzing their own learning needs, making choices about priorities and sequence for learning, and experiencing active outcome oriented learning activities. They use the resources within the Learning Resource Center so that they

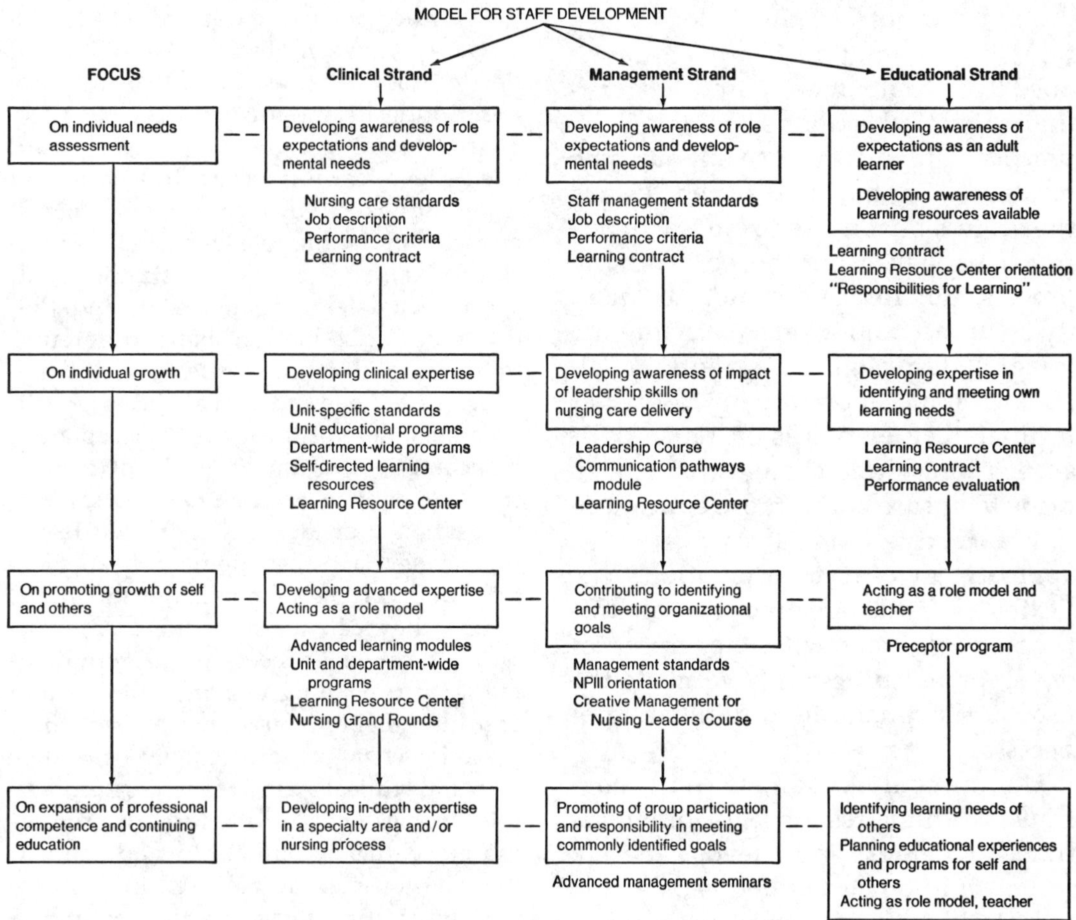

Fig. 3 Model for staff development, updated

may be comfortable in continuing to use the resources when they are fully practicing professionals on the nursing units.

Another obvious reason for development of the educational strand is that all professionals within the organization are teachers as well as adult learners. Particularly when the career focus shifts from individual growth to promoting the growth of others, the individuals may not have the skills needed to assume this role. To assist staff to become more effective as teachers of orientees, an ongoing one-day Preceptor Development Workshop has been developed to assist staff to apply principles of adult learning within the role of preceptor, to plan appropriate interventions for an orientee in each phase of Reality Shock,[3] to strategize with the orientee on how to minimize stress, and to manage conflict within the preceptor-orientee relationship.

A third development has been the elimination of the "phantom units" concept, and a complete revision of the approach to central orientation. Under the direction of Loretta O'Neill, R.N., M.S., the orientation has been developed to be competency based. Acquisition of critical skills is facilitated by practice and by the use of outcome measures. Content is directed toward the professional nurses' role at University Hospital. Concepts of nursing process, nursing care standards, quality assurance and primary nursing are integrated throughout. A central facility with skills laboratory capability has facilitated an emphasis on rapid skills acquisition. These changes have been made to ensure both a more educationally effective and a cost-effective approach to central orientation. The flexibility and effectiveness of this program together with the preceptor development program have made the use of the phantom unit no longer necessary.

Undoubtedly, changes will continue, both in response to organizational changes and needs and in response to our expanded capabilities and skills. In our attempt to promote the development of competent, confident and credible professional nurses, however, our underlying concepts remain the same.

Staff within the Department of Nursing Services are perceived as adult learners, and therefore are seen as self-directed, self-actuating individuals who can identify and meet their own learning needs if given the necessary information, resources, and support. They are perceived as having a readiness to learn what is oriented toward the fulfillment of their roles, and as having learning interests that are problem-centered and that have immediate application.

Learning needs are defined as the discrepancy between observed behavior and desired behavior as identified by role descriptions, standards, and policies. The goal of learning is a change in behavior. We believe learning occurs in a variety of different ways, such as through formal classes, simulation, role modeling, demonstration and return demonstration, and self-directed learning modules, and that different individuals respond differently to different learning experiences. However, we believe individuals learn best in an atmosphere of informality, acceptance, respect, support, and freedom of expression. We believe learning to be most effective when staff identify their own learning needs, have the opportunity to practice and apply new knowledge and skills, where they can measure their progress, when they receive feedback and reinforcement for their progress, and where there are identifiable consequences for their behavior change. Development of leadership and clinical skills are seen as mutually reinforcing. Both are essential in promoting individual accountability and defensible decision-making required in a decentralized, participatory organization and in the full implementation of a professional nursing role.

A coordinated system of centralized and decentralized staff development is viewed as the most effective system to facilitate the total staff development process. Education is seen as integrated into all parts of the Nursing Services organization. A change in knowledge is recognized as only the first step towards a change in behavior, and for any change to be effective, education must be integrated and reinforced with the clinical and administrative components of the organization. The director of nursing, coordinator of staff development, clinical nurse specialists, administrative resource persons, nurse coordinators, and members of the nursing staff share the responsibility to develop and promote continuing education experiences which ensure current knowledge and practice.[4]

REFERENCES

1. Kolb, D.A., Rubin, I.M. and McIntyre, J.M. *Organizational Psychology* 2nd ed. (Englewood Cliffs, N.J.: Prentice-Hall 1975).
2. Harrison, R. "How to Design and Conduct Self-Directed Learning Experiences." *Group and Organization Studies* 3:2 (June 1978) p. 149–167.
3. Kramer, M. *Reality Shock: Why Nurses Leave Nursing* (Saint Louis: C.V. Mosby Co. 1974).
4. Nursing Services, University Hospital, University of Washington. "Philosophy of Staff Development." 1982.

Linda A. Kent, R.N., M.N.
Director, Nursing Staff Development
Division of Nursing Services
University Hospital

Continuing Education—Treatment for Outdatedness

Dorothy J. del Bueno, R.N., Ed.D.
Associate Director of Nursing
Director of Staff Education
The Presbyterian Hospital
Columbia-Presbyterian Medical Center
New York, New York

THE PURPOSE of professional continuing education (CE) is to improve the performance of those receiving the education and thereby positively affect the care clients receive, either quantitatively or qualitatively. This at least is the theoretical basis for supporting CE.

There can be no doubt that practicing professionals must update their knowledge and performance skills; obsolescence can occur extremely rapidly in today's world. Participation in CE will indeed demonstrate the professional's commitment to continuous updating of knowledge.

Does CE really affect professional practice and competence?

The question of the relationship between CE and practice is a far more important question than whether CE should be mandatory or voluntary, university-based or institution-based, for contact hours or credit.

ACHIEVING CHANGE THROUGH EDUCATION

Education means, in the narrowest sense, the transmission of knowledge and skills. In the broadest sense, it means in some way changing individuals' behavior; that is, changing individuals' performance, beliefs and values, or the depth and breadth of their knowledge and understanding.

Although teaching and learning are parallel systems, they are not the same. Teaching is a process by which individuals *may* learn. It cannot be assumed that because teaching has been provided, an individual will change. Indeed, the individual may change, but not in the direction desired.

Changing behavior, even in only the cognitive realm, can be uncomfortable and costly—costly in the expenditure of time, energy and resources. None of us welcomes psychological or physiological discomfort.

STAGES IN BEHAVIORAL CHANGE

The Awareness Stage

In order to achieve change, an individual goes through several phases or stages. The first stage is awareness, sometimes called insight. Awareness is the acknowledgment of an unfulfilled need. Individuals are aware when they become conscious of the fact that there is a gap between what is currently happening and what they would like to have happen. For instance, awareness can be the sudden realization of being overweight and needing to lose some pounds; or the sudden realization that smoking isn't good for the body and should be stopped; or the realization that job performance isn't as effective as it should be. To help individuals develop awareness or insight, educators use techniques of consciousness raising and discovery.

When individuals are aware, they become interested and want to know more about what they can do to solve the problem: "How can I learn to stop smoking?" "How can I lose weight?" "How can I deliver more or better care to patients?" Their resistance to change is somewhat lessened and they are ready to acquire information, facts, knowledge, skills and perhaps even new values. This is the time when continuing educators can best provide content.

The Interest Stage

Educators often presume that CE participants have already passed through the awareness phase and are interested in doing something about their needs and situations. This may or may not be true. Participants may have been sent to the CE program because "they need it."

This presumption is a mistake that is often made in consumer education as well as patient education. Educators assume that because patients are ill and have come into the facility for one purpose, this is the time to teach them about health, health maintenance or prevention of disease. However, clients may not be aware that there are problems beyond the immediate health problem for which they are receiving care. Therefore, in the interest phase, educators not only need to supply information, but they may also have to overcome resistance to change.

The Trial and Application Stage

After participating in a CE program, individuals decide whether or not to use their newly acquired knowledge and skills—whether or not to attempt change. It is at this trial and application stage that staff developers and continuing educators fall down on the job. To date, because of their disregard or perhaps ignorance of the importance of the trial and application phase, they have not been able to document changes in behavior of the participants in CE.

CE providers rarely go beyond the interest phase where they provide content. They rarely plan any strategies or methodologies so they can be assured that when the participants try it, "they will like it." Reinforcement and accountability are very seldom built into CE programs, and thus no change results. To date, available documentation indicates that ignoring the application phase will result in no change in behavior.

Think of what usually happens in a typical CE session. Participants attend a session of their choice (or someone else's who thought it would be "good for them"). They acquire some new facts, concepts, approaches and/or values. Perhaps they enjoy the presentation and the interaction with other participants. They may even gain enthusiasm and decide to try out these great ideas and techniques.

The participants go back to their

The great majority of CE participants really don't believe they are supposed to do something with what they learn—that they are supposed to change. And nobody really expects the participant to be different or to change the organization.

place of practice, and whammo—reality sets in. Their attempts to change their behavior or the behavior of others is met with either resistance or apathy. The pressures of the daily routine may also interfere with implementing changes. The fact is, there is no significant "other" who really expects the participants to change their practice or others' practices, so the newly acquired knowledge and behavior is extinguished. Participants may even become discouraged from attending CE activities again.

The Reinforcement Stage

The great majority of CE participants really don't believe they are supposed to do something with what they learn—that they are supposed to change. And nobody really expects the participant to be different or to change the organization. If someone did expect change to occur, the participant would be rewarded for initiating and maintaining that change.

Sad to say, most individuals don't even try out what they acquired in the education program. They're satisfied with simply being present and enjoying the program. In general, enjoyment and attendance are the only aspects of CE which are evaluated.

NEED FOR CE STRATEGIES

What will have to be done if CE is to really make a difference in nursing practice and, ultimately, client outcomes? Educators, along with service personnel, must plan for the application/trial phase. They must anticipate changes in nursing behavior and provide positive feedback for change. Participants must see the results of the change. Before sending anyone to the content sessions, strategies to implement that content should be outlined, such as deciding who should attend the program, what reward/reinforcement systems will be built in, how much time and resources will be needed, and how to remove obstacles to implementation. If the feedback during implementation is positive, if the application of the knowledge, skills or values brings rewards such as pleasure or gratification, then learners will internalize the acquired knowledge, skills and beliefs into their practice.

Perhaps there should be a lot more programs which participants cannot attend without their boss or the supervisor who will reinforce the desired behavior change. For example, staff nurses would bring their head nurses; head nurses would bring their supervisor or department head. That way, both would hear the content and both would know what has to be done to effect change.

Marketing

Those in CE should take courses in marketing and selling, because they often don't know how to market and sell their product and services. There is more money spent in this country on cosmetics than there is on education. Why do people buy lipstick, hairspray and hairblowers? They buy them because advertisers promise these products will make the consumer look better, feel better, be more desirable, more loved and more popular. In general, people part with their money because a product appeals to them. What could encourage individuals to participate in CE and thus improve their performance?

Updating

Strategies need to be built into CE program planning as well as content. Educators now spend a great deal of time thinking about content, but very little time thinking about how to make changes happen. They need to evaluate current CE programs, including time frame. Change takes time, so there should be more longitudinal-type programs where the learning, practice, trial and reinforcement stages of CE are spread out over several months. During these months, discussions should be held to determine whether change occurred and, if not, what can be done to make it happen.

There are many logistical problems to this approach, but unless current CE programs are modified and updated, they will continue to be ineffective. Change will not happen all at once, but educators should begin updating CE programs with such offerings as one-day, half-day and longitudinal-type workshops.

EVALUATING CE

Presuming these desirable changes have been implemented—rewards, reinforcement and accountability have been built into the CE strategy; the right people and the appropriate time frame have been selected—how will CE providers know if what they wanted to happen indeed happened?

The effects of CE can be measured by identifying changes in performance. Here, self-assessment is useful, but it is not an adequate measurement. CE providers need to evaluate change by, first, measuring and evaluating both quantitatively and qualitatively the short-term effects of the CE program. For example, is the learner using the acquired knowledge and skills? Is the nursing practice of the individual different from what it was before participation? Does the behavior last or is it transitory? Does the practitioner revert back to old practice behavior?

Long-term effectiveness—evaluated by identifying changes in client outcomes, i.e., changes in morbidity, mortality, quality of life or prevention of health problems—is very difficult and costly to evaluate and is probably a long way off. Changes in participant performance or competency can be more easily measured and can serve as a beginning, but we should make a long-term commitment to work towards measuring the effect on clients.

Measuring the Efficiency

The measurement of how efficiently the change in performance was achieved can also be used in the evaluation of CE. How much did it cost to achieve the change? Cost includes dollars, time and lost patient-care hours. Consideration of cost brings up the important question: Who pays for the CE of professionals? Does the individual participant pay or does the agency (and therefore the client) pay? Perhaps individuals should pay for their own CE.

How much does CE cost?

A common CE program approved for CEUs is one which focuses on the care of patients with coronary disease. Many of these courses include 40 or more hours of classroom time. Assuming that all the participating nurses are able to commute to the program location, the per diem cost for lunches and transportation is $5.00. Registration cost, which is underwritten by a grant, is $50.00, including coffee breaks. The employing hospital pays the learner's salary, registration and per diem cost.

Assuming there are 30 nurses attending the course, and using an average hourly rate including fringe benefits of $6.00, the cost of this single CE program is $9,300 with 1,200 lost patient-care hours. (When learners are replaced by other staff doing overtime, the cost in payroll dollars is considerably greater and the cost in hours lost to patient care less.)

Another highly probable example: A state mandates continuing education for nurses. Because of the competition among hospitals, all agencies decide to offer released time with pay to meet the CE requirement of 20 hours per year. The state has 10,000 full-time RNs. At an hourly wage of $5.00 per hour, including fringe benefits, the cost of CE in this state will be $1 million with 200,000 lost patient-care hours.

Measuring Client Benefits

Both of these costs—payroll dollars and care hours—are passed on to the patient. Do patients get their money's worth? If CE leads to changes in nursing practice and if that practice benefits patients, then patients indeed get their money's worth.

However, these are two big ifs. Whether or not CE changes behavior is related to the process of teaching and learning discussed previously. The *traditional* educational process with the emphasis on *providing* knowledge and skills does *not* change practice behavior. Program participants acquire skills and knowledge by traditional methods, but such acquisition does not by itself lead to change in practice behavior.

CE can change nursing practice only if the practitioners are ready and willing to change their practice, and if the changed behavior in nursing practice is reinforced and rewarded.

NEED FOR A NEW LOOK AT CE

Educators must use different strategies and methodologies than they have been using. They must design programs which include the employers as well as the participants in CE. They must build reinforcement and evaluation into every CE program, and develop research skills to measure patient outcomes and identify the most effective programming to achieve those outcomes.

CE can change nursing practice only if the practitioners are ready and willing to change their practice, and if the changed behavior in nursing practice is reinforced and rewarded.

CE can be effective treatment or it can be costly quackery, depending on how and when it is used. It is not a panacea or cure-all for the ills of nursing practice. Rather, it should be considered a prescribed treatment for outdated practice and knowledge. Like most prescriptions, CE, in order to be therapeutic, must be used judiciously for the right symptoms and taken according to directions.

Continuing Education: Current Contradictions in Inservice

Mary Mundinger, M.A.
Instructor
Graduate School of Nursing
Pace University–Briarcliff
Briarcliff Manor, New York

THERE WAS A TIME when a relaxed, solvent atmosphere in hospitals allowed for expansion of learning activities encompassing orientation and continuing education (CE) for advanced or new practice. CE, provided by a nursing service department, has undergone a number of changes and new expectations in the past few years.

In the past, inservice was based primarily on "medical" conditions and the nursing care needed to successfully support medical care. Today, patients' hospital stays are shorter, demanding quicker and more knowledgeable nursing care. In addition to fulfilling their supportive role, professional nurses are now expected to provide "health" care.

Consciousness of the expectations of professional nursing grew about the time federal legislation forcing medical peer review and financial savings for hospitals made its impact on

This article is based on the author's study/research/experience as Manager of Nursing Service Education, United Hospital, Port Chester, New York.

Consciousness of the expectations of professional nursing grew about the time federal legislation forcing medical peer review and financial savings for hospitals made its impact on the health care scene.

the health care scene.[1] As nursing began to feel its professional value and power, it quickly became apparent that strong, creative educational efforts were needed to prepare nurses for their new effectiveness.

GROWING EDUCATIONAL RESPONSIBILITIES LEAD TO CONFLICT

Educational efforts to prepare nurses for full professional practice and to improve their practice outcomes began to appear in baccalaureate programs and were validated as consumer and nurse expectations by appearing with startling regularity in nursing practice acts being revised everywhere.[2] The only lag in the system was with the already-registered nurses practicing without access to educational programs which would upgrade their patient care.

Although inservice educators were aware of these growing educational responsibilities, these expectations were incompatible with the medical paranoia and fiscal crunch hospital nurses were experiencing. Nurses demanding recognition as professional peers with diagnostic and therapeutic powers was enough to send physicians looking for their captain-of-the-ship doctrine. In addition, national health insurance proposals and the malpractice insurance premium escalation led to widespread medical concern.

MORE TUITION-BASED EDUCATION

Cost containment legislation aimed at lowering health care costs has overburdened hospitals with operational budget cutting.[3] When costs have been cut to a minimum and the choices are then to cut further or to generate more revenue, it makes administrative sense to increase the productivity of the present educators by making some programs pay for themselves through tuition-paid attendance. This allows for growth or maintenance of educational services while decreasing costs.

As other, less visionary, hospitals cut their educational staff, more tuition-based attendance and more sharing of programs between hospitals can be expected. The hospital conducting the program has the advantage of choosing the content to be covered and increased employee morale as a result of offering the CE program at *their* hospital.

NEED FOR EVALUATING CE

The education staff must be aware of the need to evaluate their activities in terms of increased health outcomes for patients. Educators became aware of the need for stating (and achieving) behavioral objectives in their educational programs in order to justify their own activities (and salary).

Somehow, we inferred that new nursing behaviors would mean better patient care. Although that inference is borne out in many cases, educators must go one step further and identify the patient health outcomes that will occur as a result of CE for nurses. This expectation places an added burden on inservice educators.

To understand the current contradictions in inservice education, we should look at the increased focus on health outcomes for measuring educational effectiveness, and then look at the time and continuity it takes to plan and measure those outcomes. The current explosions of new knowledge needed for competent clinical care and the decrease in educational personnel available are additional factors leading to a high degree of frustration for educators. Many of the well-planned, well-needed educational ventures are interrupted to meet even more pressing needs.

AN EXAMPLE OF CONTRADICTIONS IN INSERVICE EDUCATION

What happened because of conflicting and overlapping needs at United Hospital, a recently studied 40-bed medical/surgical unit, is an example of the current contradictions in inservice education. The medical-supportive care and professional nursing care needed by the patient population in this study demanded an intense nursing education program.

Cardiac Monitoring in the Medical/Surgical Unit

A year ago, it became apparent that patients recovering from a myocardial infarction (MI) could benefit from cardiac monitoring in the post-CCU period since: (1) leaving the security of constant supervision and CCU care as well as the security of cardiac monitoring in the unit added to the anxiety of post-MI patients when they were transferred to a medical/surgical unit; and (2) monitoring in the convalescent phase of care could alert nurses to potentially lethal arrhythmias before the patient was in a crisis.

In planning for the telemetry service, we addressed patient objectives, staffing, training, medical direction and criteria for patients to be admitted to the service. Four beds out of 40 on the med/surg telemetry unit would be targeted for telemetry.

Our objectives were to increase the security level of patients leaving the CCU (as measured by verbal response, sleep patterns, calls for assistance) and to identify and treat potential cardiac complications through telemetry monitoring before clinical manifestations were present.

The staffing levels would change in order to initiate this new service, but the increase would be in the CCU, not the telemetry unit. The plan for telemetry reading was to have a monitor visible at the telemetry patient's bedside, at the telemetry unit nurses' station and on the console in the physically adjacent CCU.

Initially, the CCU nurses would be responsible for "monitoring the monitor" and for alerting telemetry nurses of a potential problem and responding when necessary to that patient's bedside. Telemetry nurses would also be watching the monitors and identifying potentially troublesome arrhythmias. Telemetry nurses would rotate with CCU nurses on a one-to-one exchange on a regular full shift basis to continue their ability to identify arrhythmias and to allow the CCU nurses to become familiar with the needs and problems of monitoring and caring for convalescent MI patients.

TRAINING PROGRAM

In planning the training program for nurses, we decided that a full CCU course would be appropriate so that the nurses would know the full scope of potential crises. However, time limited us to an abbreviated course, and we limited the objectives to the identification and anticipation of arrhythmias.

The clinical specialist assigned to this project is very patient-centered, and was concerned that we might focus nurses too strongly on the mechanics, or the little blips on the monitor rather than on the patient. She has designed and given a course that utilizes telemetry patterns as an adjunct to clinical observations and physical assessment skills. When the participants first became aware of the meanings of certain arrhythmia patterns, they gravitated to the monitor when an interesting pattern occurred. But the clinical specialist was not there to interpret; she was with the patient! It did not take long for the message to be relayed: "Go to the patient, not the monitor."

Not only are the nurses learning to correlate specific monitor patterns with given clinical signs (pulse, BP, anxiety, lung sounds), but they also begin to *anticipate* cardiac irregularities on the basis of physical findings, and to begin appropriate therapy *before* the monitor shows an ominous pattern.

IMPLEMENTATION

With an already established CCU medical board, the telemetry service fit very easily into that decision-making group. The cardiologists will make the determination of which patients will be placed on telemetry, and patients admitted to the service will be only those at least three days after a confirmed MI.

We were concerned that bed unavailability in the CCU or patients who might be medically unstable as a result of other problems would result in telemetry admissions for which we were not prepared. Here, we had a well-planned background for a continuing education endeavor. We blocked out participant and clinical specialist vacation time so the education could be accomplished and implementation of the service achieved before other programs or absences could conflict.

STAFFING PROBLEMS

However, part way into the telemetry course the NCs in both the CCU and the telemetry unit resigned, and new replacements were hired. Eight nurses in the ICU-CCU staff resigned, and their replacements were not CCU qualified. Therefore the backup in CCU for telemetry was compromised.

Although we did not have the educator staff to immediately begin a coronary care course, some of these new CCU replacements joined the telemetry course. The telemetry course, which until then had been given at times during the participants' working day, were now scheduled after working hours to accommodate the CCU nurses. This resulted in some telemetry nurses missing classes. We therefore shortened an in-depth orientation for new graduates we were piloting in order to assign that instructor to meeting the learning needs of the new CCU nurses. We extracted them from the telemetry course and tried to recoup our progress there. Meanwhile, staffing shortages began to occur in the telemetry unit, and their training schedule fell behind.

Initiation of the Telemetry Unit

A large block of vacations scheduled to follow telemetry training were now coinciding with the implementation week. Reassessment with the coordinator of the telemetry unit and the clinical specialist lead to a decision to meet the objectives of identifying lethal arrhythmias before opening the telemetry unit, but to have the physical assessment skills needed for anticipatory care taught in the weeks immediately following initiation of the service. Even though we were still (barely) able to meet the training needs, the staffing levels in both units were down more than had been anticipated, and telemetry and CCU nurses could not be utilized in an exchange. We took our group of new graduates, whose in-depth orientation had been interrupted, and brought them as staff to the telemetry unit for the remaining three weeks of their orientation so that the telemetry nurses could rotate to CCU. The orientees were supervised by the clinical specialist and given instruction on priority setting and physical care of the acutely ill patient.

Continuing concerns about adequate staffing to monitor the patients on telemetry led us to another backup proposal. A concurrent educational offering in our department has been a refresher course to recertify our volunteer ambulance emergency medical technicians in cardiac care. Recognizing lethal arrhythmias is part of their refresher course requirement, which they have successfully demonstrated. The telemetry equipment for their ambulance is still on order, so in order to maintain competence, and to assist us in monitoring the telemetry patients, we are asking them to volunteer their time during our busiest hours to watch the telemetry monitors. The CCU still holds the responsibility for this service, but these dedicated and competent EMTs are providing us with a safe backup.

This three-month period of shifting plans and priorities is just one example of the kinds of flexibility *and* accomplishment that are demanding of today's CE efforts in an inservice department.

LIMITING EDUCATIONAL PROGRAMS

The criteria we now use to determine when educational programs can be shortened or eliminated are as follows:

1. Those programs which are necessary for safe care come first. In the telemetry example, it is recognition of lethal arrhythmias.
2. Once a safe level of competency has been reached, we attempt to achieve an *improved* health outcome for patients. In the telemetry example, it is physical assessment for anticipatory care.
3. Once an improved health status is achieved, we attempt to provide terminal objectives of health maintenance and self-care. In telemetry, this would be the patient education encompassing self-monitoring of exercise, diet and recognition of potential illness indicators such as pain, edema and tiredness.

If a program must be interrupted, we have to ask ourselves some questions before ending our efforts: (1) What is the minimum objective we must achieve? (2) Have we reached it? (3) How can we maintain that basic competency until we can return to continue our progress?

We also need to ask ourselves as educators and administrators what determines an interruption in a planned program? Patient safety does; timing of a new service does; staffing does. The other factor which will always present itself is whether or not the participant will use the new skill. In times of tight educational resources, we must make top priority the teaching of skills or concepts that will be used at that time by those participants. Education for interest only can be motivational and a method of decreasing turnover, but it's a luxury we cannot afford if education for patient safety would therefore become compromised.

Now that we have devised programs for CCU and telemetry nursing competencies with limited and terminal objectives, we are ready to offer them to other nurses in the community, for a fee. We will have provided a quality offering to our staff and others, and maintained a balance of payments to allow our staff to develop other needed courses. Meeting limited objectives, defining the three-level objectives we want to meet, and determining criteria for our priorities has helped our inservice educators do two things: meet the im-

Fewer educators and higher client and administrative expectations demonstrate the contradictions in inservice today. The challenge is to do more for patients with fewer staff who must be productive, flexible and creative.

mediate and critical learning needs of the staff; and maintain a system of goal accomplishment.

Fewer educators and higher client and administrative expectations demonstrate the contradictions in inservice today. The challenge is to do more for patients with fewer staff who must be productive, flexible and creative.

REFERENCES

1. Brueckner, S. H. and Blair, E. "Cost of Education in a Department of Nursing Service at a University Medical Center." *Journal of Nursing Administration* 7:3 (March 1977).
2. "Practice Acts Expand Role of Nurses." Special Report. *RN* 38:8 (August 1975).
3. Somers, A. R. *Health Care in Transition: Directions for the Future* (Chicago: Hospital Research and Education Trust 1971) Chapt. 4, p. 39–72.

Index

A

B

C

D

E

F

M

N

Q

R

S

T

U

V

W

Y

Z